TRENT DALT(

'Kate Fisher, you are doing such in
a national treasure.'

HEDLEY THOMAS

'Kate, your podcast is excellent! Your personal connection
to these stories allows you to tell them with extraordinary
intimacy.'

HUGH VAN CUYLENBERG

'Kate, you've been inspired by Marleigh but you are
helping so many other people. It's incredible to know
that one blood donation can save three lives. I think if
everyone knew that more people would be likely to do it.'

SAMUEL JOHNSON

'You can't save cancer patients without blood donations!
Thanks for the reminder that we all have gold in our veins
that can save lives. You are reminding people of that.'

FIONA REIWOLDT

'Maddie's dying wish was to educate people about
donating blood and blood products.'

ANJ MIDDLESTANDT

'We have a saying at Missy's donors that we are saving
the lives of people whose names we will never know and
whose faces we will never see. That's so empowering.'

MILKSHAKES FOR MARLEIGH

KATE FISHER

With love

Kate Fisher

x x

KMD
BOOKS

A catalogue record for this
work is available from the
National Library of Australia

National Library of Australia Catalogue-in-Publication data:

Milkshakes for Marleigh/Kate Fisher

ISBN: 978-0-9925884-7-2
(Paperback)

Note to the reader:

The pink and black zebra in the cover art is a depiction of rare diseases (if you hear hoof beats, don't look for zebras!), Marleigh's obsession with her daily strawberry milkshakes and an encouragement to 'have a milkshake for Marleigh' when you donate blood.

This book is a collection of Australian tales of survival thanks to blood donors. It is compiled from interviews I conducted for the Milkshakes for Marleigh *podcast. It is based entirely on the recollections of recipients and their loved ones and is not intended to be represented as medically correct.*

DEDICATION

Marleigh Jessica Fisher was named M J Fisher, in loving memory of her grandpa, Murray Joseph Fisher. A proud Indigenous Tasmanian and blood product recipient, who lost his battle with melanoma in 2015, the year before Marleigh was born.

The Milkshakes for Marleigh blood donation advocacy movement was founded to address persistent critical blood shortages in Australia. It has grown to be a community of donors and recipients all over the world. Marleigh's story has encouraged people to donate the blood that has saved, prolonged and improved the quality of countless lives all over the world.

Marleigh will be reliant on blood donors for the rest of her life to provide the treatment that is lifesaving when she relapses and life-preserving for every infusion in-between.

For Andriana Koukari, because without you there may never have been a Fisher family x

And for Benjamin, Emma, Declan, Ella, Millan, Summer, Freja, Amelia and Frankie – I wish that blood products could have saved all your lives, keep playing on those rainbows until we get there x

CONTENTS

PROLOGUE

On 14 May 1984, I was born prematurely at Blacktown Hospital, NSW, weighing just over 2kg (4lb 6.5oz). On that day the lives of both my mother and me were in danger. Growing up, I remember hearing stories of my dramatic premature birth, my mother's bed rest in hospital from week twenty-nine to thirty-three of her pregnancy, her waters breaking at thirty-four weeks, her inability to feel her uterus contracting despite the monitoring equipment suggesting otherwise and my emergency C-section delivery after twenty-five hours of labour. I recall being a small child and hearing her tell stories of the obstetrician telling her that her 'uterus was flapping like a plastic shopping bag and so difficult to sew up' her recollections of 'bags of blood' going into her as she bled on the operating table.

At the same time, I was a 'tiny, bruised and battered baby' fighting for survival in a humidicrib in the neonatal intensive care unit (NICU). Premature babies frequently require blood products as they suffer from anaemia, lacking red blood cells as they are not yet ready to make their own. I was being fed donor breastmilk through a naso-gastric tube, threaded through my nose and directly into my stomach as I had not yet developed my suck reflex due to my early arrival and I was too weak to even latch a bottle. Breastmilk is much easier than formula for premmie babies to digest and protects their vulnerable immune systems from infections. I was unable to maintain my own body temperature or blood glucose levels. I needed oxygen therapy. And none of this would have helped had I not had the support of the blood products donated by my fellow Australians (likely donated before I was even born!).

As my mother and I were concurrently receiving blood products, she was begging to 'see my baby'. My mother had suffered pregnancy loss before my birth and was determined to see the little person she had grown inside her. She managed to convince a nurse to wheel her bed to the NICU, as she was still incredibly unwell, and her earliest memories of me are watching multiple humidicribs swirling around the room as her eyes played tricks on her due to the heavy pain medication and her significant blood loss.

Had it not been for the Australian blood donors who saved our lives nearly forty years ago, my family would not exist. My brother, Jake (who I mention in Chapter 3 with Samuel Johnson), and my sister, Jess – my best friends in the whole world – would never have been born. My nieces and my nephew (all of whom I'd gladly give my life for) would never have existed. I would never have met my incredible husband Geoff and had our beautiful children: Thomas, Campbell, Benjamin and Marleigh. Marleigh's chocolate Labrador seizure response and autism assistance service dog, Paddy, would be supporting another family and there would be no *Milkshakes for Marleigh* podcast. I would not be a blood donation advocate and we would not have saved over five thousand Aussie lives through our recruitment of blood donors.

Whether you make an appointment to donate blood as an act of kindness, to make yourself feel better or as a tool for virtue signalling through your social media accounts, you are doing so much more than saving the lives of three fellow Aussies. This book documents the incredible things that blood product recipients have gone on to do with their lives, the things they have achieved and the contributions they have made to their communities and impacts on the creation of future lives. The butterfly effect of one Aussie booking in (and turning up!) to make a blood donation and the impact that has for generations to come. And of course, the opposite is also true. What if you made the appointment but didn't attend, meaning someone else didn't get their time in the chair that day, and the blood supply was missing the blood products for three Aussies in need?

I created the *Milkshakes for Marleigh* podcast and blood donation advocacy movement in response to the consistent critical blood shortages experienced in Australia in 2020 when our daughter was receiving intravenous immunoglobulin infusions (IVIG) every two weeks to keep her alive. We could never look further than two weeks ahead and felt powerless in our hope that people would donate enough blood in that time to keep her alive.

In this book, Marleigh's story is woven through the remarkable stories of others who have benefitted from the blood, plasma and platelets donated by the kindness of Australian blood donors. You will read how close Marleigh has come to death on a number of occasions and how for her, IVIG made from donated human plasma is lifesaving for her when she has an acute autoimmune encephalitis relapse and life-preserving for every infusion in-between. Meaning she will be dependent on Australian blood donors for the rest of her life.

Marleigh is now seven – she became unwell at the age of three, had her first life-threating status epilepticus seizure at the age of four and commenced IVIG while in the paediatric intensive care unit at Sydney Children's Hospital, Randwick, in June 2019. In the lead-up to the first anniversary of her becoming a blood product recipient, I wanted to celebrate her survival by doing something positive to thank the thousands of blood donors who had made the donations needed to save and preserve her life. My initial aim was to get one hundred blood donations in one hundred days for the newly created Milkshakes for Marleigh Lifeblood team. Local small business owner Rick Mier, from Ricks PaintPlus Canberra, heard about my project through my social media and gave the campaign a kickstart by offering his employees an early knock-off on a Friday if they used their paid work time to make a blood donation in the morning. They all had a 'milkshake for Marleigh' afterwards at the Lifeblood centre in Garran, Canberra. This act of generosity attracted local Canberra media attention, and before I knew it, the little request that I shared on my personal social media account grew! It became a truly national campaign with hundreds of new blood donors recruited in those one hundred days, in every state and territory in Australia and with donations of whole blood, plasma and platelets. I saw the incredible power of telling Marleigh's story in encouraging new blood donors and the Milkshakes for Marleigh blood donation advocacy movement was born.

You will read in Part Two of Marleigh's story that she very nearly didn't make it to the one-year anniversary of her first IVIG treatment and that COVID-19 precautions meant that I had to say goodbye to her with the understanding that she may die in an isolation room with only the company of strangers in head-to-toe protective equipment.

In 2019, early in the COVID-19 pandemic, Marleigh was at her most severely immunocompromised. When I asked her paediatric immunologist how worried we should be about the virus and what impact it may have on Marleigh, the advice was:

'All indications are that Marleigh's immune system would not cope well with COVID-19. If she presents to an intensive care unit and she is one of two patients who need a ventilator, there may only be one available. They will look at Marleigh's medical history and give the ventilator to the other person. As a family, you need to keep this at the front of your minds with any contact she, or other members of your household, have with the community.'

This was still early in the pandemic and there was still a significant shortage of medical supplies, personal protective equipment and ventilators. But a decision was made for my husband to commence working from home and our older sons, Thomas and Campbell (who were seven and nine at the time), to complete their schooling from home. This was long before working from home arrangements, school closures and lockdowns in Australia. It was just what we needed to do to keep our precious little girl safe.

Our medical teams decided in June 2020 that it was no longer safe for Marleigh to not have a local paediatric intensive care unit (PICU). Canberra didn't have a PICU and she'd been airlifted from the Canberra Hospital to the Sydney Children's Hospital, Randwick, three times in eleven months, in far from ideal circumstances. Although it was mid-pandemic, we needed to move to keep her safe.

We moved to the Sunshine Coast, Queensland, in September 2020 into a house that we had purchased sight unseen, but just seven minutes from the Sunshine Coast University Hospital which has its own PICU and is an easy road transfer to the Queensland Children's Hospital (SCUH), Brisbane, should Marleigh ever require it. She had two admissions to the PICU at SCUH in November 2020 for status epilepticus seizures. When we moved, Marleigh was mixed-use in a wheelchair and learning how to use a speech device to communicate due to the damage autoimmune encephalitis had inflicted on her little brain. We purchased our house based on the fact that significant modifications had been made by the previous occupant who was a wheelchair user.

As this book is released, we've now lived in Queensland for three years, and our family is thriving! Marleigh is seven and is living an incredible life. Usually flanked by Paddy, she is attending school part-time, she walks (runs, skips and dances!) and speaks independently, no longer requiring the use of her speech device or wheelchair (that's due to her incredible hard work in her rehabilitation program). She has the most beautiful, fiercely protective cohort of students around her at school and is deeply embedded in our school community. She has found a true love of yoga and is happiest in a circle of crystals, meditation and yoga mats.

She uses every available surface in our house to create her art, crafts and slime, and I am forever finding her giving plastic toys and figurines a 'makeover' by painting them with my nail polishes. She's come out of her *Paw Patrol* phase and is now deep in *My Little Pony* and loves to explain the differences between 'unicorns, alicorns, earth ponies and Pegasus' to anyone who will listen to her. She is also very keen to demonstrate her 'sneaky ninja skills' due to a recent fascination with the *Teenage Mutant Ninja Turtles*.

Her brothers are the centre of her universe (bringing her the greatest of joy, humour and frustration), her daddy is her truest love, the creator of fun, wonder, magic and her biggest fan. And I am her mumma. Her safest space and the one who knows her the best because I've been to all the darkest places with her, have been her fiercest advocate, her greatest supporter through her medical journey, rehabilitation and disability diagnoses.

We don't know what Marleigh's future holds. There are some things that will never change. Ehlers-Danlos syndrome, autism spectrum disorder, MODY2 diabetes and functional neurological disorder have no cures, just treatment plans. She is currently in remission from seronegative paediatric autoimmune encephalitis and not currently on a regular treatment protocol – but she may relapse tomorrow, never or somewhere in-between. We know that she will spend a lifetime dependant on Australian blood donors to save her life if she relapses and prolong it for every infusion in-between.

I will continue this work in blood donation advocacy and know every day that there are lives saved and Aussie families that get to go to sleep at night-time together because of this work that I do. I feel deeply honoured and grateful to everyone who shared their story with me for this book and for the *Milkshakes for Marleigh* podcast.

The next book I write may be called *Milkshakes for Jake*. You will read in my chat with Samuel Johnson in Chapter 3 that last year my brother Jake was diagnosed with lymphoma. His firstborn was just two years old and his wife was weeks away from giving birth to their second daughter. This year, he completed his treatment but within weeks of his gradual return to work and just as he was about to holiday in Fiji to celebrate his remission, Jake was given horrific news. 'Relapse diffuse large cell lymphoma requiring salvage therapy and transplant.' There is no doubt that this time around he will be dependent on Australian blood donors to preserve his life, give him options for treatment and give his family hope.

To the blood donors who saved my mother's life (and likely mine too as a premature baby), to the future donors my brother will need and the thousands of plasma donors who have saved and preserved Marleigh's life, thank you.

If you have ever been a blood donor, you could have been the one to save, prolong or improve the quality of the life of one of the people in the pages of this book. They speak for all recipients when they extend their gratitude for your incredible, selfless gift.

If you are eligible to donate and never have, please consider it.

If you are unable to donate but have purchased this book, shared one of the Milkshakes for Marleigh social media posts or downloaded and episode of the podcast – thank you for joining me in my blood donation advocacy.

And if you are a blood donor – thank you not just for keeping

Marleigh alive, but for keeping a daughter with her parents and a little sister with her big brothers. I hope that within the pages of this book you find that gratitude and praise you deserve, even though I know that's not the reason that you donate. And next time you are at a donor centre, please have a 'milkshake for Marleigh'.

CHAPTER 1

THE FISHER FAMILY

As each year draws to a close, our family looks back and reflects on how lucky we are to be together – minus Benjamin, of course, Campbell's identical twin brother who died in-utero. The Fisher family story is stranger than fiction. Built on a foundation of the great love that Geoff and I share, navigating life together as a family with additional needs, who share a shopping list of diagnoses of various complex and life-threatening health conditions, alongside various physical and neurodevelopmental disabilities.

My infertility from endometriosis meant that we never really expected to be able to have children, and my infertility has been one of the greatest blessings in the challenges we have faced, because it has put everything else into perspective. We are so incredibly grateful to have these children!

It was a Saturday morning in early 2023 and our ten-year-old son Campbell was playing in a soccer carnival. He loves the idea of playing soccer and enjoys it when he gets there, but like me, he is not a morning person and it had been a struggle to get him up and out of the house in time for the first of the five games they would play that morning. As soon as there was a break, I headed straight for the little coffee van. Standing in line with the other caffeine-craving parents, I was scrolling through my phone when I saw message from our twelve-year-old son Thomas' AFL club that the father of one of Thomas' teammates had passed away. He'd exhausted all treatment options and died from an aggressive form of leukaemia following a diagnosis of lymphoma the year before. I scrolled through the photos of him with his family. Snapshots of him with his loving wife and two teenage children in the happier days before his illness and then in the days before his passing. I immediately shared the link to the GoFundMe page through the Milkshakes for Marleigh socials and also asked anyone touched by this post to make an appointment to donate blood. As while this family had just been torn apart by cancer, they'd had the options of surgeries and treatments, had their time together prolonged and the quality of that time improved by Australian blood donors. This family could lay their loved one to rest knowing that treatment options had been exhausted.

The soccer carnival was buzzing with whispers of this sad tragedy. Many families, like ours, have kids who play AFL and soccer on the adjoining fields. Local communities in Queensland share a deep sense of connection and loyalty – sport is like a religion up here and sporting clubs protect and champion their members with an enthusiasm I've never before witnessed at any junior or community level before. Think of the Queensland Maroons supporters that you see at Suncorp Stadium on State of Origin nights

— it's that level of pride and patriotism mixed with a love for their children, and that's the sporting communities in Queensland.

I heard a lady further up in the coffee line talking about how sad this man's passing was and mentioned that she was a blood donor. Laughing, she said, 'I usually really only do it for the snacks but when you see a story like this it really brings it home.' Unable to stop myself, I approached her and thanked her for being a blood donor; I explained that her donations could be the ones that have saved the life of our seven-year-old daughter Marleigh. I explained that she will be dependent on blood donors for the rest of her life, and I asked if she was okay with Marleigh coming over to say thank you. While shocked at my forthright-ness, the lady was lovely and later accepted a hug from Marleigh as she said, 'Thank you for my plasma.'

I felt her eyes on us as we sat on the sidelines, fold-out chairs and picnic blankets aplenty, watching our sons verse each other at the soccer carnival. While our interaction was brief, I feel like the gravity of our gratitude was conveyed more by watching us together as a family rather than in our brief chat. As without Australian blood donors, Marleigh wouldn't have made it past the age of three. She wouldn't get to sit and play with her toys, watching her brothers play sport, drawing pictures of unicorns and eating snacks in the sun while having snuggles from her sei-zure response service dog, Paddy. Australian blood donors don't just save lives, they keep families together, be this by saving a life or simply prolonging it, improving the quality of what time people have in some cases merely by hours to give loved ones a chance to say goodbye.

As we drove out of the sports grounds, I looked at the families in cars lined up in front of us and wondered how many of them were blood donors. Wondered how many of them knew that statistically at least one person in each of those cars would be dependent on blood donors during their lifetime. One in three Australians will need blood products at some stage in their life and yet only one in thirty eligible Australians donate.[1] I've never found an Aussie that doesn't think that donating blood is a good idea and yet so few of us make it a priority until we have a loved one who needs blood products. And I wonder if this is because the process is so anonymous. We never really know where our blood donations go. But what if there was a way to bridge that gap of anonymity between Australian blood donors and their recipients? Would that encourage more Australians to donate?

If you have ever been a blood donor, you can read the stories in this book and wonder if you were the one who saved, prolonged or improved the quality of life of the person in each chapter. You may learn the vast range of uses for blood products and you will certainly read some incredible stories of survival along the way. Many of these stories have been told on the *Milkshakes for Marleigh* podcast, however there is something new in each one that wasn't shared in its podcast episode. Many members of our community are donors to the Milkshakes for Marleigh Lifeblood team but not all are fans of podcasts! This book has been written in response to those many requests to have this available in a written format. Whether you are a blood donor or recipient, a grateful loved one of someone who has needed blood products or you are just here for some great

---

1 health.gov.au/topics/blood-and-blood-products/blood-and-blood-products-in-australia

Aussie yarns, I welcome you to the Milkshakes for Marleigh community.

With love,

Kate Fisher xx

Founder, Milkshakes for Marleigh

Host and executive producer, *Milkshakes for Marleigh* podcast

Blood donor, TEDx speaker

Blood donation advocate, storyteller and changemaker

CHAPTER 2

MARLEIGH'S STORY - PART ONE

Seems only fitting that we open this book with the kid who started this whole thing, our little lady Marleigh Jessica. She has been surprising medical professionals right from the time of her conception. Our previous children had been conceived via IVF due to my stage five endometriosis. At the time of Marleigh's conception, we had four-year-old Thomas and two-year-old Campbell. My husband Geoff and I had spent years in an excruciating emotional wrestle about what to do with our final frozen embryo. Our previous pregnancy had been a single frozen embryo transfer that had resulted in identical twin boys. Our Benjamin died midway through the pregnancy and Campbell was our survivor. I carried them both to term and birthed them both. Their pregnancy and birth was such a mix of grief, love and fear. I honestly didn't think I had the strength to try again. However, after the passing of my father-in-law Murray to melanoma in 2015, we decided to have one final shot and do one final IVF cycle.

If you know someone going through fertility treatment, please treat them with extreme kindness, respect their privacy but offer respectful support. IVF is financially, physically, mentally and emotionally brutal. Managing this final IVF cycle while working in the public health policy development for the Commonwealth Department of Health and juggling our energetic two- and four-year-old boys (who were yet to have their neurodiversity diagnosed) was a massive challenge! But dealing with the brutality of finding out as I was being wheeled into theatre to be sedated for my embryo transfer that we couldn't proceed, having the IVF clinic not tell us the truth about why and fighting to unveil the truth that the clinic had lost and 'at their best guess destroyed' our final frozen embryo that they 'can only assume mistakenly ended up in a sharps bin on a piece of equipment and was never actually frozen' actually shattered us.

And so, we grieved with rage at the IVF company for betraying our trust and not being truthful until they had their 'legal speak' locked down. We'd had IVF cycles not work before, embryos that didn't survive the defrosting process, so many early miscarriages, but this one hit differently. Thomas, Campbell and Benjamin were all conceived off that IVF cycle, in the same dish, on the same day. It's difficult to now look at my living children and not think about who that embryo could have been. And the last thing that I thought about before going under the anaesthetic for my hysterectomy at age thirty-four (surgery number fifteen – to relieve some symptoms of endometriosis and to cure my adenomyosis) was, *What if they find that last embryo and I no longer have a uterus?* The thought of getting a call from the IVF clinic one day to say that our embryo has been found or that is has mistakenly been transferred into another woman haunt me.

A few weeks after this I was deeply miserable, bloated, nauseous and exhausted. Stricken with how deeply unfair it was that despite being unable to proceed with the IVF cycle, I was still suffering from the side effects of the hormone injections. Tearily, I left my desk at work because my breasts were so sore that I was struggling to type. I remember the exact moment that it occurred to me that I might in fact be pregnant the quick count back, the realisation that my period hadn't yet arrived, the realisation that my acne may not be premenstrual and/or due to the emotional binge eating that I had been doing the few weeks prior.

I went directly to a pharmacy and bought pregnancy tests. Then I berated myself all the way back to work for putting myself through considering this as a possibility. Our fertility journey was over. There were no more embryos left and we didn't have the means or desire to start the whole process again. My husband Geoff was still deeply in shock and grieving the loss of his father earlier that year after spending the previous six months by his dad's side at every possible opportunity through his diagnosis, surgeries, chemotherapy and palliative care. So, I didn't tell him about the pregnancy tests I had purchased. We hadn't used any contraception for the previous eight and a half years because we didn't think that we needed to and that hadn't resulted in any babies so what were the chances that this would be the menstrual cycle that resulted in a pregnancy?

Thirty-two weeks later, the precious Marleigh Jessica was born. Not just our ridiculous surprise naturally conceived pregnancy, but a GIRL! Her pregnancy was by far my most gruelling – managing hyperemesis gravidarum alongside type one diabetes, while managing national sexual health policy in a Commonwealth public service role and having two spirited little boys at home felt, at times, impossible. Having a car accident towards the end of the pregnancy put an abrupt end to the working part, though. Reducing the stress in some ways but increasing it in others. Her birth was so unlike my others, and it's hard to imagine after birthing the twins, with only Campbell surviving, that any birth could be more difficult, but for so many reasons hers was. And just like everything else in the last seventeen years, there is no way that I could have done it without Geoff by my side, holding my hand, being the gatekeeper of my physical and mental space. I didn't know then how many times we would need that unconditional love and trust in each other's intuition as we made the decisions that could save or end Marleigh's life in the years to come.

From the jolt of the forceps yanking her from my body with no more pain relief onboard than a quick injection of local anesthetic and the sheer exhaustion of pushing for hours and hours, dislocating my coccyx and tearing my pelvic floor muscles and leaving me with levator ani syndrome, post-obstetric pudendal neuralgia and post-traumatic stress disorder (the combination of which would result in my invalidity retirement from the Commonwealth Public Service) to the fact that Geoff announced 'it's a girl', this birth was so different to the boys. But all such powerful experiences in the preparations for the challenges we were about to face with her health.

I'll never forget the feeling of her slippery, swollen, bruised little head and cheeks on my left breast as we both lay there in shock. Too dazed to ferret for a nipple as Campbell had (which was a total shock to me as Thomas had been born prematurely and taken straight to NICU) and just lay there wide-eyed. Looking to me to welcome her to the world. As soon as the boys were born, they felt separate to my body, but she just felt like an extension of it. And even now I struggle feel that she is completely separate to me.

Today, in late 2023, at the age of seven, she sleeps in our bed most nights; she now calls it 'the nest'. She's forever fighting sleep. We know that this is partially due to the years of intravenous steroid infusions to reduce the inflammation on her brain that have destroyed her natural circadian rhythms. But I also wonder if it's her body subconsciously trying to protect itself. All of her most serious, life-threatening status epilepticus seizures have started while she was sleeping. All have started as non-convulsive. So, while she looked still and sleeping, snoring peacefully, seizure activity was in fact ravaging her brain and causing damage. At her worst this was happening most days and in the brief periods that we had out of hospital we required hospital-grade pulse oximetry monitoring her when she slept. Just to make sure that heart kept beating and she continued to breathe through the night. That didn't always happen.

Her longest seizure went for thirty-nine hours.

Our longest hospital stint was seven weeks, in a different state, away from her daddy and brothers.

She's had three emergency airlifts in helicopters as our local hospital (Canberra Hospital) didn't have a paediatric intensive care unit (PICU).

She's had six stays in PICU, and all have been life-threatening.

For nineteen months she has double doses of intravenous immunoglobulin infusion (IVIG) every fourteen days. This required three nights in hospital at a time. Three nights in, nine nights out – and that's if she was stable. For reference, the standard protocol for IVIG treatment is a single dose every four weeks, for up to six months.

Marleigh's eventual diagnosis was seronegative paediatric autoimmune encephalitis, confirmed through proteins in her cerebral spinal fluid and abnormal conversion of glucose in her brain on PET scan. As well as neurological and seizure symptoms, lack of response to anticonvulsant medications and the only thing that had any positive impact being IVIG, which is a solution of human plasma proteins with a broad spectrum of antibody activity. It is prepared from large pools of human plasma collected from thousands of plasma donors.

Marleigh was diagnosed with a condition with no cure that was threatening her life. No amount of medical science, technology or medicine was able to stop the progression of her disease. But Australian blood donors did. As we had it explained to us: 'For Marleigh, IVIG is lifesaving when she relapses and life-preserving for every infusion in-between.'

The plasma of hundreds of thousands of Australians would be 'floating around' inside our little girl. And I can't help but compare that to the Australian cultural idiom of 'mateship'. Surely nothing feels more Australian that donating blood and that product being used to keep another Australian alive? Marleigh is still alive today because of this incredible selfless gift, and we live in hope that should she relapse again, there will be enough plasma in the pool for her treatment.

A whole other book could be devoted to Marleigh's story of survival. However, these key moments in Marleigh's survival give a sense of how incredibly lucky we are that she is still alive.

In July 2017, Marleigh was diagnosed with type one diabetes at seventeen months old. Her four-year-old brother Campbell was diagnosed forty-eight hours later. Their six-year-old brother Thomas had been diagnosed six months earlier. Luckily, we had an amazing paediatrician and paediatric endocrinologist who recognised that having three type one diabetic kids joining the type one diabetic mother in one family was highly unlikely. Over the following year, blood samples were sent to a specialised testing facility at Exeter, UK, and returned a result of maturity-onset diabetes of the young, variation two (MODY2). We are yet to find another family in the world that looks like ours.

Mid-late 2018: Marleigh went from being a happy, placid healthy baby hitting all her developmental milestones to extreme tantrums and anger. Screaming in agony without warning and without any obvious reason for pain or terror. Then there were the vague episodes where it appeared that the lights were on but nobody was home.

Initially, Marleigh's psychiatric decline (at the time I described these outbursts as being like 'daytime night terrors') were explained away as being a result of blood glucose fluctuation from her diabetes, the 'terrible twos' and worst of all 'her mother's anxiety'. But what began to follow were prolonged periods where she would appear to be in a deep sleep, completely unrousable and sometimes associated with jerking of her body and limbs. On presentation at hospital, I was informed that 'she was just asleep' and questions around my mental health and support networks were again asked.

Following a series of these episodes, I began to record Marleigh's blood glucose and ketone readings. There was a clear relation in abnormalities during and immediately after these episodes, and we were referred to a paediatric neurologist for assessment. By chance, we already had a relationship with a neurologist who was based in Sydney, as he was overseeing the management of the pineal cyst on Marleigh's oldest brother Thomas' brain.

I took Marleigh to the appointment in Sydney, and rather than driving home to Canberra that afternoon, we were admitted straight into hospital for an overnight electroencephalogram (EEG) test that measures the electrical activity in the brain using small metal electrodes attached to the scalp. A video camera was set up to film her for the night and recordings were taken over a twelve-hour period. This resulted in a diagnosis of epilepsy, and Marleigh was immediately started on medication.

The following months were filled with a desperately unhappy little girl, who was constantly suffering recurrent urinary tract infections, gastro and other viruses. Our teams kept promising us that once we found the right dosages and the right medications for her that things would get better.

January – April 2019: Marleigh was having seizures daily, followed by prolonged unresponsive periods that we later recognised as postictal periods. We started to recognise the seizure phases, which for Marleigh looked like this:

1. Prodromal and/or aura phase.
   - Becoming very clingy and anxious.
   - Lack of balance and coordination.

- Behavioural changes and extreme mood swings.
- Fatigue.
2. Ictal phase.
   - Lack of response to any form of stimulation, even pain.
   - Twitching of the left side of her mouth.
   - Twitching of arms and occasionally legs.
   - When conscious, a sense that 'the lights were on but nobody was home'.
3. Post-ictal phase.
   - Lack of response to any form of stimulation, even pain.
   - When conscious, muscle weakness and extreme fatigue. Floppy like a ragdoll.
   - Often did not recognise familiar people.

Marleigh had spent months in and out of hospital with no additional diagnosis. She was on three preventative anticonvulsant medications with a seizure response plan and yet her epilepsy remained refractory. In one of our ambulance rides in May 2019, Marleigh began having a convulsive seizure en-route to the hospital and this was stopped by an injection of a seizure rescue drug called midazolam.

From this night, her fine and gross motor skills started to significantly regress. She developed a tremor that meant raising a spoon to her own mouth became impossible. While still able to mobilise, she became fatigued very quickly and we noticed significant cognitive decline. During this time, she had further EEGs, a lumbar puncture to test her cerebral spinal fluid and an MRI under general anaesthetic to see if she had a brain tumour.

Apart from detecting inflammation in her body and recognising that her seizures did not respond to anticonvulsant medications in the way that would be expected, there were no further answers, and we could see that our child was slipping away from us. It's hard to articulate the powerlessness that Geoff and I felt in that situation.

In May 2019, we called her eight ambulances (her final count for ambulance rides in 2019 was twenty-seven via road and two helicopter rides). Most paramedics called her at a GCS 3 on arrival and raced her straight into a resuscitation bay at the hospital. GCS 3 is a rating on the Glasgow Coma Scale. This denotes a patient who is does not open their eyes (even in response to painful stimuli), makes no sounds and makes no movements. It is associated with brain injury and poor chance of recovery. The incredible team that regularly staffed the resuscitation bays in the emergency department of the Canberra Hospital got to know Marleigh and her seizure plan very well during that time. To the point that they just started stocking the right size needle to access her port-a-cath (which Marleigh still affectionately refers to as her 'special button') so that one didn't have to be tracked down in the paediatric department on arrival, wasting precious seconds.

On 28 May 2019, life as we knew it would change forever. On what was expected to be a short-term hospital stay for her under observation following an ambulance ride for a seizure that we didn't feel comfortable managing at home, Marleigh deteriorated terrifyingly rapidly. Walking across a room, she suddenly lost her sense of balance and became so ataxic she stated walking into walls and fell headfirst into a cupboard. Her vision became compromised, and she began to see double, only able to focus by closing one eye. Her speech became slurred and her demeanour reminded us of a drunk teenager. She was like a child that we didn't recognise. It was beyond terrifying. At this point we begged and pleaded to be transferred to Sydney.

What followed was two weeks of back-to-back seizures and a child who could no longer lift a spoon to her mouth due to the spasmodic tremor, and beyond our comprehension, things went from bad to horrifyingly worse.

On 10 June 2019, during a status epilecticus seizure, Marleigh needed a rescue drug called phenobarbitone. She had never had it before and she reacted badly, no longer able to maintain her own airway or breathe for herself. Our beautiful baby ballerina was intubated and ventilated.

The Newborn and Paediatric Emergency Transfer Service (NETS) helicoptered an emergency medicine doctor to retrieve Marleigh from the adult intensive care unit in Canberra and transfer her to the paediatric intensive care unit in Sydney. Initially we were bound for Westmead, but the neurologist who had been seeing Marleigh privately and diagnosed her epilepsy also saw patients publicly through the Sydney Children's Hospital, Randwick, and at his personal request she was transferred to SCUH, PICU.

Geoff and I watched on helplessly as eleven cannula attempts failed (the veins in her little arms were all stripped and collapsed from months of infusions of seizure rescue medications) and a femoral line was finally stitched into an incision in her groin. This would serve her well in the days to come as she had up to seven intravenous anticonvulsants running into those lines as we watched on helplessly as her little body continued to convulse in that PICU bed. *Note: If I was to ever have another daughter, I would call her Sascha.*

We took the advice of the intensive care team when they asked us to step outside while she was intubated, and during that time it was explained to us that Marleigh's life was in very real danger and that only one of us could go in the helicopter with her. I've never loved Geoff more than when he gifted me that time with Marleigh, without hesitation, a completely selfless act to gift those hours with her to me, if she was not to survive the night.

Seeing her baby body moving robotically with the ventilator for the first time was a feeling of shock that I will never forget. She looked like a mannequin, a robotic doll that was imitating my daughter. And even if she was to survive this night, I understood the likelihood of brain damage, and in that moment a part of me accepted that if that little girl under all the medical equipment lived, she would not be the same girl we'd once had. If she ever did open those beautiful blue eyes again, I couldn't imagine that I'd ever see them sparkle in the same way they once had.

The chopper ride was a mixture of adrenalin, shock and pain. I was only a few months the other side of my fifteenth surgery for my endometriosis and adenomyosis, a hysterectomy at the age of thirty-four. The recovery from which was far from ideal as I was on constant seizure watch and 'sleeping' in random chairs in hospitals. I'm sure that I was not yet meant to be jumping in and out of helicopters. But focusing on the piercing pain in my own pelvis gave me something to hold onto. Something that felt real in the surreal experience that I was living. Many a time I've also bitten the inside of my cheek to draw blood. The taste of the blood gave me something to focus on, to anchor myself to reality when the terror of my surroundings become too much during Marleigh's medical journey.

After we landed in Sydney, I remember sitting in a cold, brown, plastic chair while they stabilised her. The PICU doctor told me that at the onset of Marleigh's 'drunk' phase she had likely suffered a stroke and that on top of that she has now been in status epilepticus for more than thirty-nine hours. Given that her stroke hadn't been treated at the time of onset, her presenting deficits were now likely permanent. Marleigh was booked in for an emergency MRI with contrast the next day and she was placed into an induced coma. I was given a key to a little room up the hallway with a bed and told to sleep. I was speechless (maybe for the first time in my life) and I obeyed. (Months later, when I was unpacking a bag, I found a card from an organisation called Rio's Gift, who had paid for my accommodation in the hospital that night. I was so grateful to have been gifted a few hours' sleep by a fellow PICU family.)

I was back at Marleigh's bedside by dawn. Geoff was waiting at the Canberra Hospital for some images of Marleigh's brain to be uploaded on a disc as the attachments were too large to send via email (these things just seem absurd on reflection). My mum was on her way to care for Thomas and Campbell.

I learned that for one hour every morning, all parents must leave the PICU while the doctors do their rounds, and in that hour, I went in search of coffee. There was a TV mounted on the wall next to the hospital cafe and I stared at it blankly, deeply in shock as I saw the advertisement that The Wiggles would be visiting the Sydney Children's Hospital PICU that morning as part of the Sydney Children's Hospital Foundation Gold Telethon fundraiser. My first reaction was excitement as Marleigh LOVED Emma Wiggle! Then sadness for the poor families that I saw footage of in the advertisement. And then it dawned on me that our daughter was upstairs in a PICU bed fighting for her life, in an induced coma, on a ventilator. We WERE one of those families, and I couldn't have known that when they brought her out of her coma the following week, she would even recognise me as her mother, let alone know who Emma Wiggle was.

Over the next six days, in that PICU isolation room, we saw hundreds of staff. We had emergency medicine doctors, neurologists, endocrinologists, immunologists and the genetics team all looking after us. And the most brilliant and terrifyingly skilled nursing staff.

We signed a consent form for a genetic genome sequence and staff were called in over a long weekend to conduct it in a record time of five days. As I signed the form, I saw that it had been approved as it was deemed that Marleigh was 'at risk of imminent death'. The results of which gave us no further clues. Nobody could tell us what was wrong with our precious girl:

- A stroke was ruled out.
- Neuroblastoma was ruled out.
- A brain tumour was again ruled out and still the markers on her cerebral spinal fluid showed inflammation and an abnormal level of B cells.
- Swelling on her brain that ravaged her little body with seizure activity and left her unconscious for hours at a time.

The head of the PICU asked for our consent to try treating Marleigh with a high dose of intravenous steroids and intravenous immunoglobulin infusion (IVIG). It could help with a diagnosis via treatment. If it worked, it would narrow down the list of possible causes of Marleigh's illness. The doctor had seen a similar case to Marleigh's previously and this was the treatment that worked. It came with significant risks but in the absence of any other definitive diagnosis or treatment options, I signed the consent form. I felt like I needed to finally help our little girl.

It was in this conversation that I first heard the term autoimmune encephalitis, which is an umbrella term for a group of non-infectious, inflammatory central nervous system diseases. These disorders typically involve subacute, progressive neuropsychiatric symptoms with associated cognitive dysfunction, movement disorders and autoimmune seizures. One of the treatments available, especially when seizures are resistant to anticonvulsant medications, is IVIG – which has the ultimate goal of normalising a compromised immune system. It is a solution of human plasma proteins with a broad spectrum of antibody activity. It is prepared from large pools of plasma collected from thousands of blood donors and is prescribed under very strict protocols for patients who need replacement of antibodies and with autoimmune disorders.

Put simply – it was suspected that Marleigh's immune system was wrongly identifying her healthy brain cells as foreign and attacking her brain – this is what was making her so sick. If a trial of IVIG was successful, it would help to treat her condition and also narrow down a more specific diagnosis.

During this time, we had also given our consent for additional cerebral spinal fluid to be drawn during a lumbar puncture to be sent to specialists around the world as Marleigh's case had been presented to an international panel of specialised physicians. Samples had been sent to Los Angles and Berlin in the hope we could find a diagnosis, treatment and/or cure.

The best medical brains and technology across the globe were trying to find a cure for Marleigh, but in the end, it was the kindness of anonymous blood and plasma donors who gave our little girl a fighting chance. From that first IVIG infusion there was an improvement, and we finally had a treatment path and protocol.

Regular IVIG and methylprednisolone (steroid) infusions were the only thing that kept Marleigh from having constant and life-threatening status epilepticus seizures. The protocol is to have a single dose every four weeks. For a nineteen-month period, Marleigh needed a double dose every fourteen days. This would mean three to four days out of every fortnight in hospital. Then ten days out and then back in again. And this was when she was at her most stable.

We spent months on and off the paediatric neurology ward of the Sydney Children's Hospital, Randwick (shoutout to the epic teams of C2South!), and had fortnightly hangs with the paeds high care team at the Canberra Hospital (big love, ladies, you got me through the toughest time, and Claudia – we owe Marleigh's life to you and your eyebrows xx).

During this time, we also faced the decision about what to do during Australia's worst bushfires of January 2019, which burned close to our hometown of Canberra. While everyone was packing bags in case they needed to head to evacuation centres, we were checking roads to see if we could get to Sydney. The risks that we weighed up were:

• Marleigh's seizures can be triggered by heat, and she had

lost the ability to regulate her own body temperature. What would happen if we lost power and couldn't have air conditioning?

- Marleigh required hospital-grade pulse oximetry monitoring to alert us to non-convulsive nocturnal seizures. There is a back-up battery option, but if we lost power this was limited.

- Marleigh was severely immunocompromised and was not even able to share a room in hospital, and this was during the COVID-19 pandemic before any vaccines were available. Sharing amenities and sleeping in an open-air room of an evacuation centre in a setting like a school hall could result in her contracting a virus (even gastro or a normal cold or flu virus) that would be life-threatening.

- The Canberra Hospital is a tertiary referral hospital that services the Australian Capital Territory but also south-east New South Wales. It was likely that those injured by the bushfires would be flown into the Canberra Hospital, putting further strain on an already stretched health system.

- Given that Canberra had the worst air quality of anywhere in the world, there was concern about what air of that quality could do to the lungs of our immunocompromised child. And between fires and air quality, the blood donation numbers had dropped, resulting in critical blood shortages. And without donated human plasma, there is no IVIG, and IVIG was the only treatment that was able to preserve Marleigh's life.

This consideration of risk is something that won't be unfamiliar to anyone who is at the helm of a family with additional needs. Constantly making risk assessments and advocating for the best outcomes for your child. But one thing that I had no influence over was how many people volunteered to donate the plasma that was keeping our daughter alive. Autoimmune encephalitis has no cure, so that was never an option. But symptoms can be managed and quality of life improved with use of immunotherapy.

***

Marleigh's first airlift opened our eyes to the reality that our daughter was suffering a life-threatening condition; her second airlift made it feel real. In November 2019, I was in a helicopter accompanying Marleigh who was being airlifted from the Canberra Hospital back to the Sydney Children's Hospital at Randwick. She was in and out of status epilepticus and on a very slippery slope back to where she was at her sickest. Unable to last more than a few hours without seizure activity that left her unresponsive for up to six hours at a time.

Within ten minutes of the helicopter taking off, Marleigh started to vomit. She then had a tonic clonic seizure that dropped her oxygen levels dangerously low. The emergency medicine doctor administered two rescue medications and they didn't work. She was unresponsive and being suctioned so that she didn't aspirate her own vomit. I was asked to decide whether to administer a new medication because 'you know her best'. In a far-from-ideal situation, giving her a new medication in the air for the first time, I gave my consent, with little other option other than to sit and speculate about what damage the seizure may be doing to her brain.

Our pilots were trying to get up to Sydney as quickly as possible. That was when the turbulence started as we hit the smoke from the bushfires. I never again want to feel terror like I did that day. Being thrust around in the back of a helicopter, with my unresponsive three-year-old, and looking out the window to realise that visibility is poor because we are surrounded by smoke. Feeling like every decision I made could impact the long-term ability, disability, life or otherwise of my precious child.

We landed at the Sydney Children's Hospital onto the helipad that I became way too familiar with in those years. Back to our amazing emergency medicine, neurology and immunology teams (and the amazing C2South support crew!) and with some tweaks to medication, this time we were only there for weeks rather than months. During that time, I got to know families who didn't get to take living children home. I am so conscious of this every time I walk Marleigh out of a hospital following an admission. I always do it with such gratitude for the thousands of Australian plasma donors, who I will never meet, who took time out of their day to donate the blood that we need to keep Marleigh alive.

CHAPTER 3

SAMUEL JOHNSON

Samuel Johnson is an actor, philanthropist and co-founder of the charity, Love Your Sister (LYS) which is 'Australia's hardest-working cancer vanquishment charity'. Samuel is also Gold Logie-winning actor and was named Victorian Australian of the year in 2018.

'Donate blood, just donate blood! By donating you help people with all kinds of things! There is a very certain percentile of people who will get cancer but there is a much greater percentile of people that will need blood. If people donate blood, they help them all.'

Since its inception in 2012, LYS has raised $16 million for medical research and has a village of one million people who are united in their quest to vanquish cancer with hard science and the best new technologies. Samuel is also an Aussie pop culture icon – he's been on our screens for decades, and whether you struck a liking for him for his portrayal of Evan Wilde or Molly Meldrum while he was *Dancing With the Stars* or unicycling around Australia raising money for cancer research, so many

Aussies have an affection for this lovable Aussie larrikin.

In March 2023, I sat on the steps of the Powerhouse in Brisbane and interviewed Sam. He was on tour, promoting his latest book, *Dear Lover,* and I attended his event and negotiated a fifteen-minute interview with him at the end of the night. That was then reduced to twelve minutes. Primarily because Sam had spent two hours after his show signing copies of the book for each of the five hundred guests that evening and he made every one of them feel seen, heard and understood. They each left feeling like the most important person in the room.

I learned so much from watching Sam, sweating away in the Brisbane heat, the way that he engaged with the cancer patients hiding their bare heads under scarves and hats, scalps balding from the side effects of chemotherapy, to the way that he greeted the children who thanked him and turned away to bury his head in a box of books and silently weep and wipe away tears after they walked away – before a lighthearted joke about his *Secret Life of Us* character Evan Wilde and then the complete change in demeanour, the dropping of his voice a few octaves and the setting of his shoulders, masculine energy aplenty, when a corporate guest would approach.

Having watched this chameleon perform onstage, and then with the guests who had lined up for hours to get their few minutes with him to tell their story, I wondered how much would be left for me by the time we sat down to record an interview for the *Milkshakes for Marleigh* podcast. When my time came, he'd evidently thought he was finished for the night. He'd signed his books, someone had done a Maccas run and he'd chugged a few bourbon and cokes to get through the last hour of book signings. He saw me loitering and offered a polite wave, one that indicated he was done with the signings and the photos. I smiled apologetically and said, 'I'm guessing that you are wishing you hadn't offered to record a podcast interview at the end of tonight's event …' It took Sam a moment for the penny to drop and then he kicked right back into gear. He told me we needed to record backstage, I explained I had all my equipment here and that we just needed a quiet table, he looked me dead in the eye and said, 'No, I NEED to go backstage.' And in a blur of the LYS staff trying to explain that they were locking up the venue and that he had gone hours over time, I found myself running backstage and through the dressing rooms of the Powerhouse in Brisbane, for Sam to grab us a few drinks and set us up on the steps outside, on the Brisbane River, to record an interview for the *Milkshakes for Marleigh* podcast.

What do you say to the philanthropist and Gold Logie-winning actor, bereaved sibling and self-appointed vanquisher of cancer? Especially when you have a mother who has beaten breast cancer and a brother who is currently undergoing chemotherapy and fighting lymphoma, while his wife cares for their two-year-old and six-week-old daughters?

Well, first, you give him a minute, and before you hit record, you tell him that you have recognised his level of cognitive fatigue. You explain that you have a daughter who, like Sam, has a brain injury and is now living with a functional neurological disorder following autoimmune encephalitis.

I told him Marleigh's story and explained the nature of the para-social relationship that I've had with him for over two decades since the TV show *The Secret Life of Us* premiered in

Australia in 2001. I don't think it's an accident that I grew up to marry and create a family with a writer with scruffy brown hair, who is a hopeless romantic and has no concept of time. Those familiar with Sam's character Evan Wilde from *Secret Life* will understand the similarities.

I told him that my mother was a breast cancer survivor from a small country town and that she was well aware of the messages of regular self-breast checks that his late sister Connie and his organisation LYS have worked so hard to ensure is at the forefront of all Australian women's minds. And maybe that contributed to saving her life.

I explained that when we finally found a treatment for Marleigh's autoimmune encephalitis that worked, regular IVIG made from human plasma donations became what was saving and preserving her life, I knew that my mission must become blood donation advocacy, because no amount of science or medicine could keep Marleigh alive if Australians didn't continue to donate blood. So, I looked to the model of the way that Love Your Sister had not just created a not-for-profit organisation to engage on fundraising and health advocacy, but they had also created a community. And on a much smaller scale I have tried to emulate this through the Milkshakes for Marleigh movement.

And then I told him about laying on my bathroom floor, sobbing until I vomited while the reality of my thirty-four-year-old little brother being diagnosed with lymphoma sunk in. The fear that I held for him, my two-year-old niece and his wife who was thirty-six weeks pregnant. And that in those moments I'd thought of Sam and how he supported Connie. I told him that I couldn't vanquish cancer, but I could work parallel to him in the blood donation advocacy space because blood products are essential to saving, preserving and improving the quality of life for so many cancer patients.

And Sam, in all his grace, nursed a can of bourbon and coke and listened to my story. What was supposed to be a podcast interview had actually been me just spewing my story in his direction, and it dawned on me that I'd just done the same thing that I'd watched five hundred other guests at that event do. An hour earlier, I'd heard one of these guests ask Sam how he does it. How does he take on all the stories of all the Australians whose lives have been touched by cancer without being crushed by the weight of it all?

Sam said, 'Mate, I don't take it all on, all of the trauma, all of the death. But I do use it. I use it as fuel to keep going and to keep fighting. Because I don't want to see parents burying their children. I don't want cancer to keep killing people because they aren't getting the precision medicine that they need. Every cancer research institute will tell you that that's what we need to beat cancer. So, I use all these stories as fuel to give me the inspiration that I need to stop this.'

I watched another young woman tell Sam that she was recently bereaved; she'd lost her mum to cancer. She looked pleadingly at him and asked him when it would start to feel better.

Sam said, 'I'm so sorry, it's still so fresh and it's going to feel like this for a while. But I promise you I'm doing everything I can to help other families to not feel the way that you are feeling right now.'

Sam held space for these people in such a disarming way. He didn't try to sugar-coat the reality of the brutality and the tragedy of cancer. He made every person in that room feel like their experience of cancer, whether personally or as a loved one or carer, was the most important story he's heard that night, and he showed equal gratitude to the corporate sponsors and the children who put handfuls of coins into the big red fuel can that he carries around asking for donations to ensure the work of LYS can continue.

At the end of the interview, I tried to do a plug for Sam's latest initiative. Of course, these terms are always negotiated with managers ahead of the recording. But Sam shut me down told me that this interview was about blood donation. And cancer patients benefit from blood donations. He told me he was humbled by Marleigh's story and of the work that I am doing. He made me a promise that he would become a blood donor, in fact, he swore it on his late sister Connie's life. We hugged it out and then he was gone.

A few days later, Sam sent me a text message wearing the *Milkshakes for Marleigh* podcast T-shirt that I had gifted him in thanks for doing the interview. I was so touched that after all the stories he heard that night, he took the time to acknowledge ours.

These words of Sammy's have stuck with me and are such a good reminder to all advocates who often give the best of themselves in an attempt to improve the lives of others.

Sam: 'It's not necessarily about thinking that I'm changing anything, it's about knowing that I'm trying ... and I promise you, I swear on my sister Connie, that I will do a blood donation for your little girl.'

Samuel's sister Connie passed away from breast cancer in 2017. She was the recipient of many blood products during her cancer treatments. Australian blood donors prolonged and improved her quality of life, giving her more time to live by her motto, 'Now is awesome.'

Sam made good on his promise to Marleigh and made his first blood donation in September 2023 in her name. His post on his own social media accounts and through Love Your Sister read:

A little while ago I sat on the steps at night-time and talked to Kate Fisher from the Milkshakes for Marleigh *podcast about the importance of blood donation, especially in relation to cancer research and treatment. Basically, they can use every part of blood for something. The whole blood, the plasma, the platelets, the whole kit and caboodle. And there is never enough of it. Kate has a daughter who relies on plasma. Our blood is for everyone, from accident victims to cancer patients to new mums.*

I've given a lot of blood, sweat and tears for this cause over the years, but apparently, they already have plenty of the metaphorical kind. On those steps that night I promised Kate that I'd start doing my bit and I'm proud to say that I'm now a blood donor of the literal variety! It's a great way to help and it's not going to cost you a cent. And, Kate, I came good! I said by the end of the year, so I slayed it!

I was so grateful to see this announcement and it was so amazing to see the engagement from the Love Your Sister community, with renewed enthusiasm and commitments to either following Sam's lead and donating for the first time or returning to donating after a break from the blood donation chair. I hope they all 'slay it' like Sam did!

CHAPTER 4

MICHAEL KLIM, OAM

Michael 'Smash 'em Like Guitars' Klim is one of Australia's most respected sports personalities and is quickly becoming the face of blood donation advocacy. In 2020, he was at risk of losing his mobility as he was struck down with chronic inflammatory demyelinating polyneuropathy (CIPD). He is now dependent on the same treatment that saved Marleigh's life. It's all thanks to Australian plasma donors.

'When I sit in the chair and look at the bottles of IVIG knowing that there are fifty to sixty people that have donated blood for each of my treatments ... it's just staggering ... for me and for Marleigh, the positive effect it has on our lives, to continue functioning and to be a part of our communities. I was never a blood donor before this and now that I have this insight, I wish I had.'

Michael Klim is an Australian swimming legend. A triple Olympian, Klim represented Australia at the Atlanta, Sydney and Athens Olympic Games and bagged medals at every single Games totalling two gold, three silver and one bronze. When I interviewed him for the *Milkshakes for Marleigh* podcast he had just returned from a trip to the USA where he had been inducted into the International Swimming Hall of Fame. During his years of being one of the best swimmers in the world, and certainly one of the best that Australia has ever produced, he could never have imagined that he would be accepting that award aided by AFOs (ankle foot orthosis brace – a walking aid which is used to improve walking patterns by limiting movement of the lower leg which may be impacted by muscle wastage) and a walking stick. The only reason that Michael has retained this level of mobility and was able to attend the awards ceremony at all is due to the incredible generosity of Australian blood donors who have ensured blood products have been available to make the intravenous immunoglobulin (IVIG) infusions that have treated Michael's CIPD.

CIPD is an acquired autoimmune disease of the peripheral nervous system that is characterised by progressive weakness and impaired sensory function of the arms and legs. The body's immune system attacks myelin that insulates and protects the body's nerves and there is no cure. However, the progress of the disease can be slowed and quality of life for the sufferer can be significantly improved with IVIG treatment. Marleigh and Michael have used the same treatment to improve their quality of life and slow the progression of their respective diseases.

I was very nervous about interviewing Michael. A man of such incredible achievements and excellence. It was also only the third interview he had given since his diagnosis. Michael (or 'Klimmy', as he refers to himself) appeared on my screen with his trademark bald head and massive smile, and it only took me moments to forget that I was interviewing a man of such magnitude as he was so humble, kind and down to earth.

Michael described the slow puzzling onset of his symptoms in 2019. He was living in Bali and running his business in Australia, constantly travelling between the two countries as the general manager of KLIM men's skin care, and also running his Bali-based swim school, KlimSwim. He had been putting off addressing some niggling historic injuries, 'as men do', including some spinal degeneration and a left ankle injury, and he believes this may have masked some of the initial onset of the disease. However, during the rehab phase for treatment of his left ankle, Michael realised he was unable to do a calf raise on the right-hand side, this paired with the muscle weakness, impaired balance and fatigue was concerning but it wasn't until he experienced foot discolouration, autonomic sensations ('like the feeling of someone running warm water down the backs of my thighs') and severe muscle wastage, that the lengthy medical process of investigations began. It took over a year for Michael to get the diagnosis of CIDP, all the while the disease was progressing, his blood test results showing elevating protein levels due to the breakdown of muscles in his body. Michael's eventual diagnosis was CIDP, which is the long-term, chronic version of the closely related Guillain-Barré syndrome, a condition where the immune system mistakenly attacks the body.

Further complicating Michael's diagnosis and treatment was the COVID-19 global pandemic which saw most international travel cease. As Michael was receiving treatment in Australia, this meant relocating away from his children, Stella, Frankie and Rocco, who were at the time aged fifteen, thirteen and nine and living in Bali, with no clear time line on how long his treatment would last or when international travel would recommence.

Klimmy said, 'It was a year or so until we let them know of my diagnosis because we didn't want to alarm them. But now their awareness and understanding is just amazing. When we walk into a public place, they walk just in front of me or just to the left or right in case I need to lean on them … It's been a tough journey because there are a lot of things I can't do with them anymore like play basketball, surf or play tennis and that's a big part of my grieving process, no longer doing the active things with my kids.'

When he became unwell, Michael quickly realised that he would no longer be able to sustain his current lifestyle, living with his partner Michelle Owen in Bali and running a business based in Australia. He needed to prioritise his energy for treatment, rehabilitation, Michelle and his children. He told me of the relief of reprioritising his life while paradoxically grieving the loss of the future that he thought was coming in the next stage of his life. However, he does so while describing the great love and appreciation he has for partner Michelle, even if she 'got the dud version of me'. Michael shares his children with his first wife Lindy who he divorced in 2017, commencing a relationship with Michelle in 2019, well after the days of his swimming career.

As an elite athlete, Michael's experience of recovering from injuries or setbacks was structured rehabilitation programs and precise recovery time frames. A diagnosis of a chronic medical condition like CIDP offers none of this structure as there is no cure. The best he could hope for was for the progression of his disease to slow down and for him to maintain as much mobility as possible, for as long as possible. And luckily for him this was possible with the treatment of IVIG, made from the plasma of Australian blood donors.

'It's been levelling and humbling. This complete change of identity has impacted my mental state. I think Marleigh is lucky because of her age she is still learning about her condition, but I was told the stats like that 30% of people with my condition end up in a wheelchair.'

Michael's body had been his 'tool' for so much of his success in life. It is what he conditioned and trained to swim at world-record pace and to win Olympic gold medals and now it is the thing that is changing his entire life by attacking itself. He said now the most amazing thing about being part of the sport of swimming has been the community that has rallied around him, particularly Daniel Kowalski and Ian Thorpe and how important the bonds that they forged during their time in the pool have now become to him in this time of need. He had this message for Australian blood donors:

'It's very hard to put into words ... even when I sit in the chair and look at the bottles of IVIG knowing that there are fifty to sixty people that have donated blood for each of my treatments ... it's just staggering ... for me and for Marleigh, the positive effect it has on our lives, to continue functioning and to be a part of our communities. I was never a blood donor before this and now that I have this insight, I wish I had.'

In 2023, Klimmy launched the Michael Klim Foundation which will help raise funds for CIDP research and help sufferers and carers. Michael shared his story with me in the hope of thanking the thousands of blood donors who have played such a crucial role in his treatment.

He was the face of Lifeblood's National Plasma Week Campaign in October 2023, telling his story to help recruit new blood donors and thank the donors who have had such a remarkable impact on his life.

CHAPTER 5

FIONA REIWOLDT

Fiona Reiwoldt is a bereaved mum who got more precious time with her daughter Maddie thanks to Australian blood donors. Maddie lost her battle with aplastic anaemia when she was just twenty-six years old. Fiona thanks the blood donors who gave them extra days of watching TV and eating ice cream together in their PJs on the couch. She is now honouring Maddie's dying wishes and her legacy through the organisation Maddie Riewoldt's Vision (MRV). She hopes that one day nobody will have to 'fight like Maddie'.

'Maddie had hundreds and hundreds of blood transfusions, and she would not have survived without them. The only reason we had that extra time with her was because blood donors took that hour out their lives to donate blood ... Maddie's first and original wish was to spread awareness about the importance of blood donation but then we realised there was just so much more to be done ... She's still such a big part of our lives.'

Maddie's parents, Fiona and Joe Reiwoldt, co-founded MRV

together in 2015 to 'honour Maddie's legacy'. MRV supports patients and families living with bone marrow failure syndromes while also raising money to fund medical research towards better treatment options and a cure. Maddie's brother Nick is a member of the MRV board, and as per Maddie's wish, they also promote the importance of blood donation.

The Riewolt family name is well-known in Australia due to the careers of cousins Nick and Jack in the AFL. Jack with the Richmond Tigers and Nick with the St Kilda Football Club and now with his AFL commentary and sports media career.

Maddie Reiwoldt was just twenty-six years old when she died from complications of a bone marrow failure syndrome called aplastic anaemia. She lived a beautiful vibrant life before she became unwell. Aplastic anaemia is a condition where your body stops producing new blood cells. This results in fatigue, vulnerability to infections and being prone to uncontrolled bleeding.

Maddie began her life in Tasmania; the Reiwoldts relocated to the mainland when Maddie was three, but Fiona says that for the Reiwoldt family, Tasmania will 'always be home' as it holds so many wonderful family memories with brothers, Alex and Nick, and their extended family, in the time before they even knew about bone marrow failure syndrome. Maddie's final resting place is the beautiful little town of Orford, on the east coast of Tasmania, as this is what Maddie described as her 'happy place'.

Fiona: 'It's rather beautiful, you drive down a section of road called "paradise", it's hilly, and you come down around the side of the river and up over the hill and I can feel this feeling coming over me and it's just one of total peace, warmth and this gentle

... healing place. It's very special to us and I have very special memories of our children growing up in Tassie together.'

As a little girl, Maddie was 'feisty, cheeky and fearless'; she was a typical tomboy, never liking dresses but with a phenomenal ability to negotiate, especially if wanting something from the shops! At nine, Maddie suffered a head injury after being hit with a shotput during a sports lesson, impacting her executive functioning and leaving her with anxiety and fear about things like separation from the family and the dark – a challenge that would impact her life in the years ahead.

After leaving the cold weather of Tasmania, the Riewoldts moved to Queensland, and Maddie enjoyed the sunshine, surfing and the beach. It was quickly realised that Maddie was an exceptionally talented sportswoman. She played baseball, hockey, AFL and soccer. The bruises on her legs from playing soccer were what first alerted Fiona that something might not be right with her daughter.

It's heartbreaking that the WAFL (Women's Aussie Rules League) wasn't active before Maddie passed away because everyone who knew Maddie says that she would have made an exceptional mark on the creation of that new league or any other sport that she chose. Her natural sporting prowess, fierce loyalty to a team (or whatever team big brother Nick was playing for!) and tenacious spirit would have made for a formidable opponent in whatever sporting endeavour she chose to pursue. But it was not to be, as Maddie's final six years were spent undergoing relentless medical interventions and blood transfusions in a fight to stay alive. While Fiona is grateful for the extra years that they had after she was diagnosed, she finds it excruciating to think of

Maddie's early twenties being dominated by her illness – years that should have been carefree and filled with fun and freedom. Her final stint in hospital lasted 270 days in an intensive care unit before her devastating passing in 2015.

Fiona: 'You learn so much going through things like this … I just can't bear the focus certain people put on such small problems … And whinging about getting old! People forget what a privilege it is to get old.'

Since inception in 2015, MRV has raised over $8.7 million and supported thirty-six medical research projects in partnership with medical research institutes, hospitals and universities across Australia. MRV has established the first Centre of Research Excellence in Bone Marrow Biology in Australia, dedicated to promoting the collaboration of expert researchers around a common purpose, and providing the technical and peer support necessary for catalysing innovation across specialisations, ideas and projects in bone marrow failure syndromes.

In addition, the Fiona Reiwoldt Nursing and Allied Health Fellowship to upskill nurses providing care for patients impacted by bone marrow failure syndromes and improve dissemination of information and education of newly diagnosed patients and their carers. The legacy of Maddie Riewoldt's life is to support other patients and their families with the resources they need to #fightlikemaddie, including blood donation awareness.

One recipient of the support from MRV is Seth. A boy from the north-west coast of Tasmania who at the age of eight was diagnosed with aplastic anaemia. One of the great challenges of being diagnosed with a chronic health condition is that close to 35% of Australia's population live outside capital cities, meaning probable challenges to accessing the medical care required. Even if you do live in a capital city there is no guarantee the specialist care you require will be available in your area. For example, we had to relocate away from Canberra as Marleigh needed a local paediatric intensive care unit (PICU) and the Canberra Hospital (in the nation's capital!) does not have one, meaning constant helicopter retrieval by the Newborn and Paediatric Emergency Transfer Service (NETS) to the Sydney Children's Hospital at Randwick where she could receive appropriate care from her neurology and immunology specialist teams in a PICU environment. Put simply, the Australian Capital Territory did not have the staff or resources to treat and keep our child alive.

Seth and his family had the same challenges with the health services in Tasmania when he became unwell. His mum Jess described the horror of what they thought was an inconvenient ongoing nosebleed transforming the young family's lives into one of medical emergency, their family being separated, first with Seth being transferred to Hobart at the other end of the state and then off the island of Tasmania and onto the mainland to receive emergency care in Melbourne at the Royal Children's Hospital. Jess speaks of the uncertainty as a formal diagnosis for Seth was investigated and their dependence on Australian blood donors at this time:

Jess: 'Seth was having daily blood tests to determine the levels for his blood and platelet transfusion. Whenever he fell asleep it was my time to cry, and I would cry every single night … I just wanted it to all be a bad dream and be over because I was so scared of what the future would look like for him.'

This is where MRV stepped in to provide education, support

and a sense of community to Seth's family. Jess explained that MRV contacted her while Seth was at the Royal Children's Hospital in Melbourne. As a St Kilda supporter, Jess already knew about MRV and was thrilled when Seth was invited to Maddie's Match – the annual AFL game between the St Kilda and Richmond football clubs that honours Maddie's memory, while raising awareness about bone marrow failure syndromes. Unfortunately, COVID-19 resulted in the cancellation of this game, but Jess speaks of how much they appreciate the support of MRV and in particular its telehealth nurse who had provided ongoing support and information.

I've stayed in touch with Jess since we recorded her podcast episode in 2021 and she is thrilled to report that Seth, now eleven, has achieved remission. He is enjoying so many aspects of an average Aussie childhood. He's back at school full-time, hanging out with friends at the beach, riding his bike and reading Harry Potter! Jess, Seth and their family thank MRV for the work that they do and Australian blood donors for keeping Seth alive. Of the blood donors who kept Seth alive, Jess says, 'It's so hard to find the words to thank the blood donors who have kept our family together. Without them I would have had to say goodbye to my little boy.'

Seth finally got to attend Maddie's Match in 2023 and got to spend time with the St Kilda Football Club, being gifted his own jersey and running out with the players on game day. This was a timely boost of support for Seth and his family as he has faced some recent setbacks to his aplastic anaemia remission and has restarted on many of the medications he had been able to cease.

Maddie Riewoldt's story was one of the most requested ones that I've ever had through the *Milkshakes for Marleigh* podcast; her story has touched so many people all over Australia. None more so than one of Australia's most loved women, two-time *Big Brother* winner, disability advocate and media personality, Reggie Bird. Reg has used her platform to open up the conversation of disability as she has shared her journey with the genetic condition retinitis pigmentosa, a degenerative condition that will rob Reg of her sight and maybe her hearing. Following her first *Big Brother* win she remained in the public arena and shared her journey of parenting son Lucas through cystic fibrosis.

Reggie shared with me her reliance on Australian blood donors during two ectopic pregnancies, having available blood products was the safety net that made her lifesaving surgeries possible. She extends this gratitude to the blood donors who gave her more time with her close mate, Maddie Riewoldt.

Reggie: 'She was a beautiful girl; I just love Maddie to bits and I miss her dearly. And the Riewoldts are just such beautiful people, just down-to-earth Tassie people ... I remember her telling me about the bruises on her legs playing soccer and then the diagnosis of aplastic anaemia but I never thought it was something that would take her life. I remember us counting down the days to her bone marrow transplant, and I can't believe she spent those seven months in the ICU and I kept flying down to see her and just after the last time I saw her was when she passed away. But she was just so full of life! Fiona sent me a text message after I won *Big Brother* again and said that Maddie would be so proud, she loved her sport but she REALLY loved her reality TV! Thank you to the blood donors who helped keep Maddie alive, I think everyone should donate if they can … And if you haven't done it, get out there next time and donate.'

Fiona still holds Reggie in such high regard and through continuing her relationship with Maddie's friends, she maintains a connection to Maddie. Fiona told me of Reggie:

'In lots of ways Reggie reminds me of Maddie. In life you just have to accept your lot and get on with it. She's one tough girl, Reg, and that's why her and Maddie got on so well.'

One of the foundations of the Milkshakes for Marleigh movement is to offer blood product recipients and their loved ones a platform to tell their stories, thank their donors and encourage new ones. I always wanted to achieve this with a focus on the positive things that recipients achieve with their lives after receiving donated blood products – be this in their careers, seeing their families grow up or with contributions to their communities. Blood donors gave Maddie a fighting chance, prolonged her life and improved its quality, and they gave Maddie and her family hope. A gift that is hard to qualify. The magic of Maddie's story is that even after her passing she is impacting on the lives of Aussies every day by encouraging people to donate blood: ensuring improvements in medical science and research and improving access to information and education for newly diagnosed patients and their families.

I thank Fiona for sharing the story of her precious daughter with me and will always think of Maddie in her PJs eating ice cream straight from the tub with her mumma, and we will visit her next time we are in 'paradise' as we drive to Oxford on our next Tasmanian road trip. How lucky would any of us be to have a family like the Riewoldts if we ever have to #fightlikemaddie?

And how lucky was Maddie and the whole Reiwoldt family to have Australian blood donors in their corner making that fight possible? Fiona says that: 'Maddie's friends continue to donate blood and send me photos of an arm donating blood, and that's so important because without it, Maddie wouldn't have had as much time, and for us, blood donors gave us hope. And I just hope and pray that people keep donating blood.'

In our chat, Fiona and I found such common ground in the experience of being mothers who have both fiercely advocated for the best outcomes of our daughters and to the AFL for the incredible support they have offered our families – the Riewoldts with St Kilda and us with the GWS Giants, particularly player Callan Ward, who continues to make our lives magical.

Fiona's final message to Australia blood donors:

'It is a gift of life that you have given, and you gave my daughter the best possible chance, and without you we wouldn't have had her for as long as we did … And for those that are considering it, what an amazing thing to say that you have done, to have either saved someone's life or given someone's family the chance to have them for longer. I will just be eternally grateful.'

CHAPTER 6

JIMMI & EMMA

Jimmi caught on fire on his second birthday. Decades later, his wife, Emma, suffered a life-threatening postpartum haemorrhage following the emergency delivery of their baby girl. The only reason either of them survived is due to the generosity of Australian blood donors. Now they get to watch their daughters grow up.

Emma: 'Our obstetrician asked me to stop trying to compete with Jimmi! He had already died three times and after I nearly died a few times he asked me to stop trying to compete with him ... For me, it was actually quite peaceful and that's how I know how close it came.'

On his second birthday, Jimmi sustained burns to 30-40% of his body; he died three times because of his injuries but was able to be revived. Nobody knew if he would survive and if he did what his quality of life would look like. When a patient suffers severe burns, plasma infusions can offer some relief by replacing lost fluids and proteins which can stop a patient from going into shock. In addition, patients may have blood transfusion requirements from surgical blood loss, reduced red cell production and increased red cell destruction. Most patients will require multiple transfusions as they recover from their initial injuries and will require additional blood products if they have skin grafts and reconstructive surgeries.

Jimmi spent the next forty years in and out of hospitals having surgeries, skin grafts and reconstructive treatments. There is no way to count how many times he has needed blood products or how many blood donors have donated to save his life. But if you have donated blood in the last forty years, there is a chance that you have been the reason that Jimmi gets to live his amazing life, love his incredible wife Emma and watch their little girls grow up.

Jimmi couldn't have imagined that nearly four decades after his initial injury, he would again be dependent on Australian blood donors. This time to save the life of his wife Emma following the birth of their second daughter, who had an emergency pre-term delivery due to the life-threatening pregnancy complication pre-eclampsia.

Severe bleeding, or postpartum haemorrhage, after the birth of a baby is the loss of more than 500ml of blood after a vaginal birth or more than 1,000ml after a C-section delivery. This level of blood loss can make mothers very unwell and anaemic making it very difficult to recover and care for their babies, and if blood loss exceeds these volumes, then mothers' lives are in danger. Emma lost over 3,000ml of blood. More than half her blood volume. Because she was so unwell, she experienced this as 'really quite peaceful' having no concept that she was having life-threatening seizures as her body began to shut down; her obstetrician described it as 'just like a tap was turned on inside you', she had no idea that her newborn daughter's life hung in the balance as she herself came so close to death.

Emma: 'In the space of six hours Jimmi came so, so close to losing his wife and his newborn daughter. We were both so close to death.'

Jimmi and Emma had gone from the young couple concerned about Emma's health and the premature delivery of their baby, but mostly excited to become a family of four and introduce big sister Millie to her new baby sibling, to Jimmi coming so close to being a widowed, bereaved single dad. How quickly the world can change in six hours.

Emma required three blood transfusions to save her life, but she survived and reflects on the joyous moments of introducing Millie to baby sister Addie. Knowing the only reason they get to be together as a family is because of the hundreds of strangers that donated the blood that saved them all.

Jimmi: 'As unfortunate as the situation is that we have been through, we consider ourselves to be incredibly lucky and are extremely grateful. Our outcome could have been so much worse.'

Jimmi is in a very unique position to comment on luck, gratitude and fortune. Without Australian blood donors he would not have survived his second birthday, gone on to meet and marry Emma and become father to their beautiful daughters. On his second birthday, while his mum was inside their house baking his birthday cake, Jimmi went out to the garage, climbed up and got some petrol, accidentally pouring it on himself. He went inside to seek assistance from him mum and at that exact moment that she opened the old gas oven, unknowingly exposing her petrol-soaked toddler to a naked flame as she removed his birthday cake from the oven. The fumes from the petrol set Jimmi alight and caused a house fire. Jimmi is incredibly grateful to not remember the experience and it breaks his heart to think of what his mother went through that day. His mother watched him die and be revived three times – at the house, in the ambulance and then at the hospital. She had to wrestle with the questions of what his quality of life would be if he did survive this horrific accident.

For the first five months after the fire, Jimmi had at least two surgeries per week – every time, he required blood products. Because of his burns, it became almost impossible to find areas of undamaged skin to create skin grafts, and because Jimmi had so many blood transfusions his body began to reject blood products. His mother described it to Emma that it was like 'Jimmi had become allergic to other people's blood'. In the end he could only tolerate plasma rather than whole blood transfusions as his medical teams fought to keep him alive. In the four decades that followed, Jimmi has spent twenty-seven out of forty years in and out of hospital having the ongoing surgeries and treatments that he needed to live a full and active life. A life that (alongside being a loving husband and father) Jimmi has dedicated to serving and protecting members of the Australian public. In the Australian Federal Police, Jimmi has worked all over Australia and overseas, working in some of the most specialist areas of policing, tackling some of the toughest physical assignments and training requirements. He has never let his injuries stop him from achieving his goals and he does not define himself as having a disability. Jimmi explains that his injuries are not limited to the external burns that people may see; he also had internal injuries. This includes damage to his lungs and vocal cords from the burns and the petrol that he swallowed when it splashed onto him. This means that overuse of his voice can result in him being unable to vocalise due to fatigue, and he also has to be aware that he only has 75% of his lung capacity, meaning that physical activity is challenging. In addition, Jimmi is unable to breathe through his nose due to damage to his sinuses from the burns. The burns have also changed his skin as it has been 'flattened like playdough' meaning it does not have the same flexibility that it did and is unable to sweat in the same way as his undamaged skin. Resulting in Jimmi being very prone to overheating as his body is unable to sweat to regulate his temperature – he is only able to sweat in patches. What defines Jimmi, however, is not his physical limitation and injuries, but his determination to achieve all of the things that he was told he could never do due to his injuries. I laughed with Jimmi and Emma as we reflected on the fact that due to his burns, Jimmi has to be extremely careful with sun exposure, has limited lung capacity, an inability to breathe nasally or to regulate his own body temperature – so his response to this is to strive for acceptance into a profession in which part of the application process and training requirements are gruelling outdoor physical assessments. I admire Jimmi's tenacity and his optimism, against all the odds, to live such an incredible, fulfilling life and I am so grateful that Australian blood donors gave him the chance to do this.

In her 'spare time', alongside her public service career and raising the girls with Jimmi, Emma is the creator of Stay Put Girls, a social media platform dedicated to encouraging women to prioritise their health and wellbeing by making time to exercise, to support their physical and mental health. Emma road-tests sports bras and creates such wholesome, relatable content about bodies of all shapes and sizes and the importance of self-love.

Jimmi and Emma are two beautiful Aussie souls who fell in love and started a family. They both dedicate their professional careers to supporting other Aussies to live their best most safe and well-supported lives. And most importantly, they approach every day so intentionally and with such gratitude for the gift of life they have been granted by Australian blood donors.

Emma is a frequent plasma donor and has been such a huge supporter of my Milkshakes for Marleigh blood donation advocacy work and she is one of the people that I think of when I speak about Australian plasma donors being the only reason that Marleigh is still alive. When Marleigh was at her sickest and there was nothing anyone could say or do to alleviate our terror (and despite the fact that we had drifted apart as we had both immersed ourselves in motherhood and our young families), Emma would often just send me a selfie or tag me in a social media post of her doing a plasma donation, *For Marleigh*. This felt like the greatest act of kindness that anyone could offer our family at that time. If you ever have family or a friend that is unwell or has a sick family member and you don't know what to say or do, I can highly recommend making a blood donation for them. You will be showing them how much you care, and you will be saving the lives of three fellow Australians.

And there could be a little girl like Marleigh, a mumma who has just given birth like Emma or a little toddler burns victim like Jimmi with their life hanging in the balance who see the light of another day, thanks to your donation.

CHAPTER 7

JOEL MASON

Joel Mason describes himself as: 'An experienced and inspirational educator, a family man, a lover of all things in and around the ocean, a blood donation promoter and a shark attack survivor.' He thanks Australian blood donors for saving his life and his leg after he was bitten by a shark while surfing in Nambucca Heads, New South Wales, while bleeding out on the sand after he was rescued from the water.

Joel: 'I realised how serious the situation was when I heard an emergency responder say the words: "If you haven't got any blood in that helicopter, don't bother coming."'

Joel Mason is a forty-two-year-old man from New South Wales, he is husband to Nicole and father to three beautiful young kids. He was the quintessential Aussie kid that grew up with a surfboard under his arm from the age of five. He is a teacher, volunteers in his local community and encourages fellow Aussies to donate blood because he knows that without the generosity of Australian blood donors, he wouldn't be alive.

In 2019, Joel was out for an early morning surf, something he has done for decades in Nambucca Heads, northern NSW. It was a beautiful Sunday morning, the surf wasn't great but with a spare hour he was making the best of the morning doing the thing he loves. He was surfing an area that the locals called the bar, in the water with three other surfers, when the shark attack occurred. Joel remembers, while admiring a pod of dolphins, he 'saw a torpedo coming and then felt the bump'. Initially, Joel was unaware of the severity of his injuries until he realised that his leg wouldn't work, and then with horror, observed a trail of blood and realised it was coming from him.

The other surfers in the water with Joel and those watching from the break wall watched the attack unfold, but it all just happened too quickly for anyone to warn Joel of what was about to happen. In some ways, Joel was unlucky that he was the one the shark chose, but without those three other surfers who dragged him ashore for lifesaving treatment, it is unlikely that Joel would have ever made it out of the water.

In another stroke of fortune, watching from the break wall was a member of the Nambucca Surf Lifesaving Club. He applied a torniquet and this slowed Joel's blood loss and bought him some time for emergency services to arrive. Joel was urgently airlifted to Newcastle's John Hunter Hospital, but before leaving the scene of his shark attack, he required an emergency blood transfusion, the first of many blood products he would need in the months to come. Joel credits his initial calm and survival instincts to a lifetime of volunteering and competing as a Surf Lifesaver both in Australia and internationally. However, the gravity of his situation hit him after this airlift in a helicopter when he found himself in an emergency department bed, staring at fluorescent lights on the ceiling and he could hear someone screaming, 'Save my leg, just save my leg,' and Joel realised it was him. He also realised how close he had just come to death and that he really wanted to live. How his life had irrevocably changed in the space of the last few hours and the life that he had known before he dived into the water that morning would never be the same again.

'It's one of those things, we are in their domain! You've got a one in 11.5 million chance of being attacked by a shark, I've spent my whole life paddling, surfing, diving and swimming throughout the world. That morning I was in such a rush to get out there and enjoy the morning that I didn't do some of the things I normally do ... that stays with me ... A friend reminded me after the attack that a helicopter had signalled us out of the same spot six weeks before and I'd forgotten about that. But Aussie lifestyle is being on the beach and such a high percentage of us live on the coast, we are in the water all the time. It's just one of those freak accidents that happen. I'm so lucky to be able to put my kids to bed at night-time, hug my wife and celebrate my birthday with friends and family.'

Joel remembers laying on the break wall and seeing faces appear as he was trying to comprehend what had just happened. A local man named Paul had been looking out into the water with his girlfriend when he witnessed Joel being attacked by the shark and ran down to help as he was pulled from the water. On the way, Paul grabbed two travellers named Luke and Cat, who had stopped to admire a pod of dolphins in the water, and found themselves administering first aid to keep Joel alive until the 'local firies' got to the scene and moved him. When they called emergency services and requested the helicopter the advice they gave was 'don't bother coming if you don't have blood'. Luckily, they had blood and Joel received his first blood transfusion at the scene of his shark attack and this was able to keep Joel alive for long enough for the helicopter to land and airlift him to Newcastle (350km from Nambucca Heads where the attack occurred), however, they needed to needed to land en-route and pick up more blood in Port Macquarie (134km down the road) to keep up with what was required to preserve Joel's life. This blood was delivered via police escort to meet the helicopter as it landed. In total, Joel received nearly four litres of blood and an additional 1.5 litres of plasma that day, and without a doubt owes his life to Australian blood donors.

Joel: 'We thank our lucky stars for so many things that day. From the people who helped me to the people who had donated blood in the days leading up to the accident. It's a miracle that I survived and maybe a bigger miracle that I still have a functioning leg!'

Joel doesn't class himself as disabled, but the function of his leg is impaired and impacted by lymphedema. He's undergone many surgeries, support from the trauma unit and an intensive rehabilitation program to have the best possible outcome. A leg that he uses to this day to continue swimming and surfing and spending time in the ocean with his kids. He's even surfed again at the exact same spot that he was bitten by the shark. He goes out with a best mate on a jet ski, and they have developed a system where he jumps off the back of the ski when the wave comes and gets picked up and taken back out for the next one. Joel is passionate about making the best of his situation despite the challenges he now faces, and he credits surfing and getting back in the water to having a huge positive influence on his mental health, something so important after facing your own mortality in the way that Joel did.

Joel: 'I grew up in a small coastal town in NSW, I spend so much of my time surfing, swimming and paddling ... as a small kid I was thrown in the rock pools, it's part of the Aussie culture and the lifestyle, it's part of everything we do! My wife and kids love the beach and it's got a real healing effect when you are in the ocean ... you get in the water and forget about all the other things you have to do. And the salt water! My wife often says, "We have to go for a salty swim!" We take the dog and the kids to the beach or lagoon and it has that healing factor.'

His greatest challenge when surfing is that he is a 'goofy footer' mean that he surfs with his right foot forward (which is the leg that was injured in the attack) so he's needed to retrain himself to surf and he describes the success as 'pretty hit and miss' but the muscle memory for surfing is coming back, he's making progress and he's so grateful to have the opportunity to be back in the water, doing the things that bring him so much joy.

'You never go in the ocean and have a bad time!'

Unless you get bitten by a shark.

'A shark attack is such a freak accident! I know for my mental health if I'm spending time in the ocean, it's a good thing! Life is busy, we've got three kids, my wife and I work, it's a twenty-four-seven world ... but when I'm in the water I get to disconnect. And it's all thanks to the people who donated the blood products I need to be able to live.'

There are so many things that Joel would never have had the chance to do if he'd died the day of the shark attack. He'd have left his wife Nicole a widow and not had the chance to partner with her in raising their three young children. He would have not been able to continue his work as a teacher, educating Aussie youth and he would not have been able to continue making contributions to his local community through his volunteer work.

Today, you can find Joel at a local high school where he provides career advice to high school students to support them in setting and achieving goals to set them up for their own life journey. One of the projects he is most proud of is his initiative to sign up students to start donating in high school with the hope that they will become lifelong blood donors. He says people call him inspirational, but he is just trying to be the best person he can be with his second chance at life, and he is in constant awe of his family and local community who continue to support him. His greatest words of affirmation, however, are for wife Nicole, who has been his greatest support.

Joel: 'I just want to take the time to thank my wife. She has been my greatest support and does such an amazing job looking after our family. I just want to be the best dad, be the best husband, be the best friend I can be if I have a mate who needs me. I just want to enjoy it all! I want to do it all with a positive attitude and a smile on my face. We are all going to have hard days, we are all human, but if you can have that positivity around you and are doing good things, hopefully that will inspire other people to do good things too.'

Joel hopes that by sharing his story he inspires people to book a blood donation.

Joel: 'I'm grateful for people who donate regularly but we need to recruit new donors. It's amazing how you can do something as simple as one blood donation and that can be split up to save so many lives. The fact that you get a text message to say that your donation has been used is such an empowering thing! You might not be the medical professional that gave treatment but being the person that took the time out of their day to donate their blood is an awesome feeling and to get that text message to say it's been used is the best "payment" you could get.

'There are plenty of people who hear my story or Marleigh's story or imagine a cancer patient that has needed blood or someone who has had an accident, and they think they should donate but don't know how. The process for registering and booking a blood donation is really easy! And it's the best feeling to know that you've helped to save someone's life.'

CHAPTER 8

GRACE JOUKHADAR

Grace is a schoolteacher, yoga teacher and spiritual activist. She is wife to Ben, mumma to Marcus, Aliyah and Raya. Raya is her youngest and was diagnosed with leukaemia just after her fourth birthday. Grace shares what it is like to parent a child with a fifty-fifty chance of survival and thanks the blood donors that made her treatment possible.

Grace: 'The gratitude I have for these absolute strangers who are donating their blood and saving my daughter, I just can't thank them enough ... Thank you to all the blood donors out there. If you want to help, please just go and donate blood. It's such a practical way to help Raya and so many kids like her who need it every day.'

In 2019, Grace and Ben decided to move their young family from Melbourne to Sydney to be closer to Grace's family. Grace and the kids made the move first, with Ben staying behind in Melbourne to finish up work and pack up their house. Grace was to settle the kids into the new school year and then they would all be reunited as a family to commence their new life in

Sydney. Within weeks of moving, they would find out that Raya was very unwell. This was further complicated by the border closures between Victoria and New South Wales due to COVID-19, meaning that nobody could travel between the two states. With Ben stuck in Victoria, Grace was told that their four-year-old daughter Raya had leukaemia.

Before becoming unwell, Raya had just started preschool. She was doing dancing and swimming lessons, playing at the park, loving art and craft and playing with her older siblings. In the year before her diagnosis, Raya's life was interrupted with an increase in illnesses. Intermittent fevers, a nasty urinary tract infection, persistently swollen tonsils that were always explained away as viral illnesses. The family were in months of isolation following the COVID-19 lockdown orders (Melbourne had the longest and strictest lockdowns in the world) and yet Raya's fevers persisted despite not having any community contact to contract a virus and in the absence of anyone else in the household being unwell. Grace knew something wasn't quite right with her little three-year-old daughter but she 'would never have suspected leukaemia'.

Grace mentioned her concerns to Raya's paediatrician in the weeks before they left Melbourne. The paediatrician ordered some blood tests as part of the handover process to her new paediatrician in Sydney. The bloods showed some inflammatory markers, but Raya was recovering from another bout of tonsilitis. Grace was given the instructions to repeat the blood test when she arrived in Sydney a few weeks later and to follow up with the new paediatrician in Sydney. This second blood test resulted in Raya being diagnosed with leukaemia.

Leukaemia is tricky to diagnose as it 'hides in the bone marrow', so even though Raya was showing signs of being unwell in the months leading up to the diagnosis, it doesn't show up on blood tests until it reaches the blood. In the weeks between the two blood tests that Raya had, the leukaemia had progressed to affect 90% of her bone marrow, and Raya was diagnosed with acute lymphoblastic leukaemia. The day that Raya was diagnosed, Grace quit her job as a schoolteacher to become Grace's full-time carer.

Grace: 'It's like you're on rollerskates, everything happens so fast. Suddenly you are told that she is diagnosed and while you are in shock and trying to deal with that and what that means and what this disease is, you are then given a treatment plan and then you are in all of these meetings trying to understand what all of this means … Suddenly it all just happens! She starts chemo! She starts steroids! She gets a central line! She goes under a general anaesthetic! It literally all just happens the next day … just so quickly. You mind can't even catch up!'

The greatest blessing of this time for Grace, Raya and their family was that the day Raya was diagnosed, the border closure between New South Wales and Victoria was lifted at midnight and Ben was on the first flight at 6am the next morning to be with his family and to support Marcus and Aliyah through their sister's diagnosis and transitions to new schools while Grace moved into the life of oncology and childhood cancer, her life now confined to the walls of the Westmead Children's Hospital in Sydney.

Raya's treatment commenced with a thirty-day induction period of steroids and chemotherapy, and she was hospitalised for the first six weeks as she didn't have any response to chemotherapy. This was terrifying as it appeared that treatment was not going to work. Eventually, Raya's body did respond, but slowly, and she was labelled as a 'high-risk leukaemia patient' meaning that in addition to the chemotherapy treatment protocols, Raya required a bone marrow transplant.

Raya was diagnosed in February 2021. She needed to be in complete remission to undergo a bone marrow transplant, however, after seven months of intense treatments and consistent hospitalisations, the bone marrow transplant went ahead in August, as nothing else appeared to be working. This had a massive impact on every member of Raya's family. Emotionally, mentally, financially and socially. While Raya was the child with 'special needs', they became a 'family with additional needs' as their entire life was turned upside-down. Particularly given the hospital visiting restrictions with the COVID-19 pandemic which meant that for the first year Grace 'barely saw [my] other children'. Grace reflects on Aliyah being so thrilled that she made it to her dance performance, relieved that 'Mummy watched me! She didn't get a call to go back to the hospital be with Raya'. The juggle of the emotional mental load of being the parent to a chronically sick child is that when you are in hospital with them you desperately miss your other children and then when you are with your other children it's so difficult to be fully present because your mind is still in the hospital room with your sick child. It's an excruciating reality shared by so many carers, and Grace shares the incredible relief of having just moved back to Sydney where her parents, sister and brothers were living and the incredible support network that was offered to them all with Raya so unwell.

The other key support that Raya had during her chemotherapy was Australian blood donors. Chemotherapy damages the genes inside the nucleus of cells; it is much less likely to damage cells that are at rest, such as most normal cells, and more likely to target growing, abnormal cells, like cancer.

Grace: 'The chemotherapy kills your cells basically, and so your white cell count drops to zero, as do your platelets and your haemoglobin, they all drop dramatically and your body is not able to reproduce them because of the chemotherapy. So, with children like Raya, who have leukaemia, they need blood transfusions to bring their levels back up in order to survive. They would die without it. She had forty-five blood transfusions in the first year after diagnosis ... Every time Raya had chemo, she needed blood products of some kind ... platelets, haemoglobin or IVIG to help boost her antibodies.'

Although she wasn't quite in remission in August 2020, Raya's dad Ben was able to donate the bone marrow that she needed for transplant. Grace describes this as her rebirth.

Grace: 'Before transplant, she never made it to remission, after the transplant she was in remission but they told me that she had a fifty-fifty chance of that working and if it didn't there was nothing they could do for her ... I can't tell you the agony and terror that was in my mind about what if she doesn't make it to remission? I'll never forget the moment that they told me that she got to remission.'

During the bone marrow transplant, Raya relied heavily on platelet transfusions due to persistent bleeding noses and her blood simply not being able to clot. The six months following Raya's transplant were so precarious as her body slowly rebuilt itself a new immune system. She was still undergoing regular hospital visits, appointments and monitoring and she needed to limit her community contact, her schooling program delivered at home by Grace, as they protected her from the threat of viruses while her body grew stronger. The first two years are the highest rate for relapse.

Raya is now two years post-transplant, she is in remission and is living a big, beautiful, fulfilling childhood! Grace shares regular updates of Raya attending school, family holidays and the incredible advocacy work their family are doing now. This has included sharing their story with Australian broadcaster Hamish McLauchlan in partnership with The Snowdome Foundation, illustrating the trauma of childhood cancer and also partnering with Adam Kennedy from the GWS Giants AFL Club, in his role as an ambassador for the Kids with Cancer Foundation.

Later this year, Grace is going to lead Raya, Marleigh and me in a yoga and meditation session where we can hold space for our shared experiences and trauma, celebrate and appreciate that our girls are still with us when so many of the families we have met along the way no longer have their children earthside and to radiate our gratitude to the blood donors who have kept our daughters alive and our families together, because without Australian blood donors, both Raya and Marleigh would no longer be alive.

CHAPTER 9

MONIQUE 'MERMAID' MURPHY

In 2014, Monique Murphy was at a university party when her drink was spiked and she fell from a five-storey balcony onto a glass roof. While she was in a coma in the week following the accident, her parents were wrongly informed that it was a suicide attempt.

Blood donors saved Monique's life and she has gone on to earn remarkable achievements, representing Australia and claiming a silver Paralympic medal in swimming and being a fierce advocate in disability and endometriosis awareness and advocacy.

Monique: 'I remember looking down at my leg and wondering why it was bandaged in a point rather than at a ninety-degree angle? Our brains are very cruel, and I could still feel my foot ...

'I have two anniversaries, the first is the accident and the other is the day we knew that I would survive ... Without blood donors there would be no anniversaries.'

Monique grew up loving swimming, she swam competitively

all through high school and had big dreams of one day representing Australia at an Olympic Games. Monique had put that dream on hold in 2012, when she was offered a highly sought-after spot in a furniture design course at Royal Melbourne Institute of Technology. With her heart still in the pool but her head telling her she needed to pursue a different career, she accepted the offer, took a gap year to travel and then moved from Canberra to Melbourne to commence her studies.

Monique's gap year was the year of the London Olympics. That year the Paralympics enjoyed increased coverage and visibility on commercial broadcast networks. But Monique missed all of that as she was 'somewhere in Spain'. She travelled and enjoyed some other freedom of her youth that her commitment to swimming had not previously allowed. She shares how many talented athletes in Australia will never reach their full potential due to the financial limitations.

Monique: 'I was feeling the pressure to travel, go to uni, to start studying and start my career … The bottom line was that I stopped believing in myself and I left my swimming career knowing that I still had more to give and I had not yet reached my full potential.'

In April 2014, Monique was just three weeks into her second year of university in Melbourne and working as a residential assistant at her university college when her life would be changed forever. She went to a party, with no intention of getting drunk, as while she wasn't rostered on that night, she was at her place of work and speaks of a culture between her and the other residential assistants of not drinking excessively at university events. While she does not remember much of the night of her accident, she remembers having one drink around 6pm and then everything goes black until she woke up in hospital a week later to see her parents standing over her bed telling her that they loved her and all she could think was, *My parents are divorced ... they don't live in Melbourne ... how much trouble am I in that they've had to come down here?*

'But I knew straightaway that something really wasn't right. I did a body scan, and I knew my spine was okay because I could feel my body and knew I was experiencing pain. I could hear and understand my parents so I knew my brain was okay, but I still had breathing tubes in as I had been on life support for a week so I couldn't communicate with them to tell them that I couldn't remember.'

Eventually, across many attempts at scrawling with a pen and paper, Monique managed to convey to her parents that she couldn't remember anything. Her parents explained to her that she had fallen from her fifth-storey balcony onto a glass roof. While memories of this time are patchy, she remembers looking down at her ankle and wondering why it was bandaged at in a point rather than at a ninety-degree angle. Her brain could still feel her foot and had not yet comprehended that gravity of her injuries. It took around two days after she first woke from her coma for her to overhear doctors say the words 'foot amputation', and her new reality started to come into focus. Monique turned to an intensive care unit nurse and asked, 'Did they cut off my foot?' just as her mum and aunt walked into her hospital room. The nurse did not respond to Monique, but instead to her mum with the simple apology, 'I'm so sorry, I thought she knew.' Monique had in fact been told many times that her foot had been amputated but the catastrophic nature of her injuries and the pain management in place to keep her comfortable meant that she had no memory. But this time, Monique remembered. Her mum explained that when she fell, her jaw had saved her brain and her foot had saved her spine. She explained that the most life-threatening of her injuries was the laceration to her neck due to the blood loss, and together they cried. While Monique didn't realise it at the time, blood donors had saved her life.

Once she understood the enormity of her injuries, Monique describes her panic being replaced with calm and a sense that 'everything was going to be okay'. She knew that with her family's support she would not be alone in her recovery or rehabilitation and that they got her through the darkest of days and biggest of challenges. Her parents and her brother made sure that she never felt alone in her struggle.

The additional trauma for Monique's family was that the police wrongly informed them, and the students at her university, that her accident was an attempted suicide. For over a week they sat at her bedside in the intensive care unit with a very different version of how she sustained her injuries. This is something that Monique struggles to move past. She just wishes that the police had waited until she woke up or had done some more investigative work at the university residential college before wrongly informing her parents that she was trying to end her life. Monique's dad's greatest fear during that week where they thought it was a suicide attempt wasn't that Monique was going to die, it was that she might wake up and be disappointed that she hasn't succeeded. Monique saw many psychiatrists and trauma psychologists following the accident and they have all ruled that she was not suicidal, and this was not an attempt to end her life. Monique strongly suspects that her drink had been spiked. There are no conclusive pathology results to confirm this as blood and alcohol tests were not done at the hospital due to the critical nature of her injuries and the attempts to save her life. As she does not remember the night (total memory loss is indicative of drink-spiking) it's impossible for her to piece together the events leading up to her accident, but she is clear that she was not depressed and not having any thoughts of self-harm in the lead-up to the accident occurring.

While Monique was not depressed at the time of her accident, she does acknowledge that she is at a great risk of having poor mental health outcomes now that she is a person with a disability. She has been proactive in managing this aspect of her health and has been working with Lifeline to help reduce the stigmatisation that she felt as a person in hospital wearing a bracelet that wrongly identified her as a *SUICIDE RISK*.

Monique decided that the way to prove to the world that she was okay was with what she did next, and she is so grateful to the Australian blood donors who made this possible. She required blood transfusions primarily to keep her alive from the significant blood loss from the laceration in her neck, which was full of glass bordering on major arteries and her windpipe, but then for her ongoing injuries and as a safety net for the eight surgeries that followed. Falling on a glass roof meant significant injuries to much of her body and for her ankle 'it looked like a bomb had exploded inside it', which also resulted in huge blood loss. Her first thought when she found out that she'd needed blood products was an extreme sense of pride as she had been donating blood since high school and was excited to be both a donor and a blood product recipient. She says of both blood and organ donation:

Monique: 'You have to be willing to donate what you have when you can because after the accident there is nothing that my family or I would have turned down to keep me alive, so we all have to be willing to do the same.'

At the age of twenty, Monique had walked away from a career as a professional swimmer, had done some travel, been accepted into an exclusive furniture design course and realised that it wasn't for her, started studying social work (off the back of a long-standing relationship volunteering for St Vincent de Paul), had her drink spiked and nearly died, had her leg amputated and learned to live life as a person with disability. And for Monique, that was just the start.

Monique: 'I hate using the word inspiring because my core purpose as a person with a disability is not to inspire people! People with a disability are a lot more than that! But I knew that sport for people with a disability is an area that needs a lot more attention and I could be a part of that movement and that change.'

Monique now has a public platform and is a fierce advocate for people with disabilities, both in and out of sport. She is passionate about informing people that the Olympics and the Paralympics are two completely different events and feels incredible frustration about the differences in funding and television coverage the two events receive. She sees this as a reflection of the value placed on para-athletes when compared with their able-bodied counterparts and she says that it makes her feel 'worth less', when her swimming races are competed during the commercial TV ad breaks or run late at night in a highlights reel, rather than receiving the prime-time commercial coverage that the Olympic swimming does.

Nine hundred days after her accident, Monique was standing on a podium at the Rio Paralympics receiving a silver medal for the 400m freestyle. Despite being concerned that she would be photographed on the podium with a 'snot bubble' (she was both unwell and overcome with emotion after the race) she describes this moment as one of deeply mixed emotions. On one hand, she was representing Australia, standing on a podium receiving a medal for her swimming achievement. Yet on the other hand, the only reason that she was there was because she lost her leg. Such conflicting emotions. And yet it was the moment she felt like she gained her independence again, something that she feels she was robbed of after her accident.

Monique: 'Swimming is my language, and this was my way of saying to my parents, "I'm going to be okay! If I can do this, I'm going to be fine with whatever I want to do." When I got out of that pool in Rio, I let go of all that trauma … That accident is never going to be a happy memory, but now we can leave it in the past, it's not something that we need to drag with us anymore.'

Today, you will find Monique working at Sporting Wheelies which is a peak body for Paralympic sports. She works to provide inclusive sports, recreation and rehabilitation therapy and with the commitment to making active goals of all levels possible for people with disability. One aspect of her job that she loves is to take wheelchairs out to schools and run wheelchair sporting events with able-bodied children to give them the experience of having a disability. She loves challenging people's perception of what it means to be a person with a disability and educating people about the vast spectrum of different experiences that description encapsulates.

She is also a fierce advocate for women's menstrual health in sport and uses her experience of having endometriosis to educate and advocate for herself and the athletes around her. She reflects with frustration the way that pain associated with endometriosis and/or adenomyosis is treated so much differently to physical injuries associated with her swimming career or her disability.

Monique's story highlights that none of us know when we will be the one who is dependent on the kindness of blood donors to survive. One day, Monique was a healthy, strong nineteen-year-old, living and studying in Melbourne and her greatest concern was planning her upcoming twentieth birthday celebrations which were only a few weeks away. Within hours, and at the hand of her drink-spiker, she would have a broken jaw, collarbone and ribs, lacerations to her neck, a torn triceps tendon, a tibial plateau fracture and the imminent amputation of her right foot. She would be fighting for her life and would not have survived had many Victorians not donated their blood in the days before her accident. To describe the life that she gets to live now, she says, 'There is a reason that I woke up!' and she is now dedicated to a life of service 'sharing life lessons, one prosthetic at a time!'.

Monique: 'To whoever donated the week before my accident, thank you, you without a doubt saved my life ... Please don't wait until you need it or someone you love needs it before you realise the importance of it, donate blood now!'

CHAPTER 10

DR DINESH PALIPANA

Dr Dinesh Palipana, OAM and 2012 Queensland Australian of the year, is a doctor, lawyer, TEDx speaker, author, disability advocate and researcher in spinal cord injury. He is the first quadriplegic medical intern in Australia and the first person to graduate as a doctor with a spinal cord injury. Dinesh and his beautiful mum, Chithrathi Palipana, are deeply grateful for the blood donors that made his lifesaving treatment following his motor vehicle accident possible. They have dedicated their lives to supporting patients and their carers whose lives are impacted by injury, illness and disability.

Chithrani: 'They were tough times and I would not wish them upon anyone. It's the love, courage, determination and hard work that got us here. We are who we are today because we never took NO for an answer, we never asked God, "Why me?" We gave what it takes. Together we were stronger!'

In the evening of 31 January 2010, the world would change forever for Dinesh and his mother Chithrani. Dinesh, a medical student, had just visited his mother and after dinner was driving home. At around 8:30pm, just north of Brisbane, Dinesh lost control of his car when it aquaplaned on a slippery patch of wet road. That night would change both of their lives. Dinesh would, among many other injuries, sustain a spinal cord injury and become quadriplegic. Chithrani would become his carer.

To spend time in the presence of these two is such a treat! Their banter is reflective of two people who feel completely safe with each other, of two people who share the special intimacy that only comes with having experienced the incredible level of vulnerability that comes with fearing that your son is going to die and then becoming his carer, advocate and greatest cheerleader in his adult life. I caught up with them at the Sunshine Coast Community Awards in 2022, where I was cheering on my incredible friend Emma Madsen who was a finalist in the awards. Dinesh and I were already firm friends; we had met doing disability advisory work and he had been a guest on the *Milkshakes for Marleigh* podcast in its first season, and I have always been incredibly grateful for his endorsements and support of my work. I had heard him speak so many times about the incredible woman that his mumma was, but to meet her was such a joy!

Chithrani is a stunningly beautiful but unassuming woman who has an air of grace and confidence that I aspire to. She knows who she is, and she is proud of that woman. But most of all she is proud of her son! Dinesh delivered the keynote address at the awards function to a captivated audience, and while Chithrani must have heard hundreds of iterations of the same speech in her years of supporting him in his disability advocacy work, she was the most captivated woman in the room.

After the formalities we had hugs all round and as I gave them giant chocolate freckles (knowing Dinesh's weakness!) for the car trip home, I introduced Chithrani and Emma. Chithrani does incredible advocacy work for carers in Australia and Emma is the founder of The Carers Club. She is best known for coining the term 'bereaved carer', a term that is being recognised worldwide as the way to describe the experience having someone that you care for pass away and the experience afterwards. More than just grief, being a bereaved carer recognises the change in identity and lifestyle that comes with the person that you care for passing away, as well as the emotional labour and mental load of tasks that need to be completed after their passing. Chithrani was enamoured by Emma and her passion for supporting carers, in each other they found a kindred spirit and it was such a special moment.

Dinesh and I stood aside and chatted about his book release, my podcast and Marleigh. He always so thoughtfully asks after my children, who all have various physical and neurodevelopmental disabilities alongside their complex and chronic health conditions. The kindness in his eyes as he asked after them made me wish so deeply that he had been one of the emergency medicine doctors that I had met in resuscitation bays so many times in emergency departments during status epilepticus seizures.

When Dinesh came on the podcast as a guest, he told me that he wouldn't change the night of his accident and that if he had the ability to resolve one thing in his life it wouldn't be to make his legs work again, it would be to cure his depression.

Dinesh: 'If someone came to me with a time machine and said they could go back in time and fix my legs, to reverse my spinal cord injury, I don't think I could do it. It's been over eleven years since my accident now … I've just come from the research lab where I'm doing spinal cord injury research, I'm hoping to change what spinal cord injury means to people. I feel like I appreciate life more now. I feel like I appreciate my mum more now, I certainly appreciate Australia more now. I know a lot of good things have come from surviving my accident.'

Dinesh's story inspires the work of Milkshakes for Marleigh so much as the focus has always been not on the trauma and the need for blood products, but the incredible lives that people go on to live, the things that they achieve and the contributions they make to their communities and in their personal lives and families that would not have been possible had someone not donated the blood that they needed to survive.

Dinesh: 'I became too aware that life is fleeting and tomorrow is not guaranteed so I need to make the most of all the time that I have.'

When I interviewed Dinesh in 2021, it was the International Day of People with Disability, and he was an ambassador. We spoke of his incredible commitment to his disability advocacy work, and I asked him what he would like the legacy of his efforts to be.

Dinesh: 'I would love to see the day when we don't need to have these conversations. I would love to see the day where we don't need to have the International Day of People with Disability … I would love to see the day when people with disability are just accepted, don't need to face all the challenges that they do and that their families are happy and comfortable knowing that their loved ones will live a safe and supported future.'

Dinesh was driving along the Gateway Motorway in Brisbane on 31 January 2010 when it is assumed that his car aquaplaned, resulting in his car to roll over. He suffered a broken neck, a spinal cord injury which resulted in him losing all function from the chest down including his fingers and parts of his arms. He does not know what medical interventions he received in the immediate aftermath, but he knows that it's highly likely he required blood products immediately following the accident or during the subsequent surgeries and treatments he had in an effort to sustain and improve his quality of life in the future.

Dinesh: 'I learned something really important about medicine in that journey. When I was in the ambulance, the emergency medicine doctor was one of my lecturers from university, so I know that he was an incredibly skilled and talented man. What I learned from that experience was not what he did, the procedures that he performed or his medical skills, it was the way that he made me feel. And what he taught me. People often don't remember the treatments they have but they do remember the way they felt at the time. I don't specifically remember having blood products, because I don't remember much at all of that time, but I strongly suspect that I would have needed them.'

Dinesh sees firsthand the lifesaving power of blood products as he prescribes them on a daily basis as an emergency medicine doctor at the Gold Coast University Hospital emergency department (ED), which is the busiest ED in Australia. He speaks of the importance of having blood on-hand for trauma patients and how time-limited they often are to give these products to patients to keep them alive. He explained that the end goal of trauma treatment is to find the bleeding and stop the bleeding, but until that has happened many patients require blood transfusions to keep them alive as they would bleed out and pass away before this treatment could be successfully completed. In addition, blood products can be used sub-acutely for patients who have been bleeding for days to weeks which can affect their organs, protect from infections and bring them back to normal to complete their treatments.

Dinesh: 'To know that we have access to blood products [in emergency medicine settings] is so reassuring … The way our teams mobilise and trust each other when someone who is critically ill or a trauma patient comes in is just incredible and it's one of the things I love the most about emergency medicine. It's such a deeply human activity, to keep someone alive.'

Before studying medicine, he completed a law degree, and I asked him if when he was diagnosed with a spinal cord injury and quadriplegia if he considered ceasing his studies in medicine and giving up his dream of becoming a doctor, but he said this never really crossed his mind, even when it was really hard and when multiple institutions suggested that him practising medicine wasn't a realistic option, because becoming a doctor was always his greatest passion and biggest dream. Giving has always been so important to Dinesh and he has realised that it is his greatest ingredient to true happiness. Cheekily, he suggests that all those who are eligible should donate blood because it might just make them happier.

'Blood is so important and donating it is the easiest way to save a life!'

Dinesh is now a bestselling author, having released his memoir *Stronger* in 2022. It's an outstanding testament to the strength of the human spirit and the strength of love in motherhood. I am so grateful that Australian blood donors played such a big part in saving Dinesh's life so that he and his mum, Chithrani, could go on to contribute to the lives of so many Australians and in support of carers and people with disability all over the world.

CHAPTER 11

MARLEIGH PART TWO - THE RELAPSE

Every time I feel the crispy coldness of a Canberra winter, watch my breath create a little cloud as I breathe out and have to factor in scraping ice from the windscreen of the car to leave the house, I will be taken back to the two separate incidents, both in June, but almost exactly a year apart when we were prepared for Marleigh's death. Both times involved a heavy fog that made landing a helicopter for our emergency airlift difficult. The first, Marleigh was taken by a road ambulance out to the Canberra airport because the Neonatal Emergency Paediatric Transport Service (NETS) helicopter wasn't able to land on the Canberra Hospital helipad due to bad weather. The second time very nearly cost Marleigh her life. When the NETS helicopter was sent from Sydney to retrieve Marleigh, the fog was so thick they were unable to land and had to return to Sydney where the team were then put into an ambulance and driven the three hours to Canberra. On arrival, they alerted the Sydney Children's Hospital to the fact that Marleigh required urgent PICU care and another helicopter was dispatched to take her to Sydney. All the while, our severely immunocompromised girl was exposed in an open-air adult intensive care bay as all the isolation rooms were being used by COVID-19 patients.

Only a few weeks before, I had been proudly sharing the newly created Milkshakes for Marleigh Lifeblood team and my campaign to recruit one hundred new plasma donors in one hundred days to help to replenish the stocks of plasma that Marleigh has required in the past year. I really wanted to use this as an opportunity to thank blood donors and to celebrate that they had gifted us a bonus year with our beautiful baby girl.

On Mother's Day 2020, I posted the following in my personal Facebook page along with some family photos:

What we have learnt is that the greatest intimacy, love and trust in a family can only come through vulnerability. And you can only allow yourself to sit in that uncomfortable space of vulnerability if you feel safe. In the safety of the love of my little family in the last year I have adored my role as a mother. We have taught each other that it's okay to fail, to make mistakes, to have regrets — because our home and our family will always be the safety net that catches us. This year, Geoff, Thomas, Campbell and Marleigh have been that for me and I hope that I am always their safe place to land. Before the last year I have always said that, 'I love being a mum, #blessed etc!' but I now know the visceral feeling of love, terror, gratitude and peace. I will love my children in all their states, and whatever life keeps throwing at us, we will make it work.

Our children embody strength, determination, humility and resilience. They came from my body, my love for them is fierce and

I am their mother.

It was chilling for me to read *I will love my children in all their states*, which at the time obviously referenced our Benjamin but almost foreshadowed the challenges that Marleigh was about to face.

In the lead-up to the anniversary of her first IVIG infusion, Marleigh had enjoyed a few months without any significant, prolonged, life-threatening status epilepticus seizures. This all changed on 15 May 2020, when Marleigh was airlifted to the PICU at SCH due to prolonged status epilepticus, which thankfully hit her while we were already admitted to hospital for her regular three-day IVIG and steroid infusion. When accessing Marleigh's port that afternoon, it had taken three attempts and a whole lot of distress; this makes Marleigh very seizure prone and within twelve minutes of falling asleep she was completely unresponsive, with pinpoint divergent pupils and rhythmic left-side face and arm twitching. This quickly progressed to a full-body tonic clonic seizure in which the oxygen saturations in her blood dropped like they never had before. Marleigh has a very strict seizure management plan that is well tested, and when it works, it works very well; when it doesn't it usually means that the status epilepticus episode is indicating an acute recurrence and relapse of autoimmune encephalitis.

On this occasion, the entire seizure management plan failed. I was beyond grateful to have Claudia as the nurse looking after us as she had looked after Marleigh through many a prolonged seizure before and I have no doubt that the precise decision-making, her crisp and confident directions to paediatricians and intensive care doctors is likely what saved Marleigh's life that night and kept her with us for at least one more sunrise. Even though the universe seemed to have other plans for her ...

Within twenty-four hours she had developed septic pneumonia and efforts to reduce her sedation and wean her out of the induced coma, with the hope that she would start to breathe on her own, had failed. As her intubation tube was suctioned, I watched the secretions go from clear, to cloudy, to yellow and thick and then to chunky and accompanied by blood clots. While her head and body burned with a fever rarely dropping below forty degrees, her hands and feet were icy cold. Her blood pressure dangerously low and unable to move the blood down to her extremities which were blue and mottled. Our girl was really, really in trouble.

On admission to the PICU, the possibility of COVID-19 testing had been discussed, but given that our whole family had been in isolation for the previous nine weeks and that she only had a very mild fever (not uncommon post-sedation or post-seizure) and no respiratory symptoms, they made the clinical decision not to do it. The doctor explained that if that picture changed then Marleigh would need to be put into isolation and we wouldn't be able to see her for twenty-four to thirty-six hours until she'd had two negative COVID-19 swabs.

It's never a good thing when an ICU doctor pulls up a chair and sits down – they usually appear and then disappear as quickly as they have emerged. Their feet barely touching the floor, let alone their bums touching a seat. On day three in the PICU, Dr Stuart concisely and yet compassionately explained to me that he now had a febrile child with pneumonia and ongoing seizures, he was left with no choice but to COVID-19 test her. But once that decision was formally made, I would no longer be able to see her. All the personal protective equipment (PPE) the staff were wearing would need to change (not significantly given that Marleigh is immunocompromised they wear most of it whenever in contact with her to protect her from acquiring anything from them). He said that he was about to 'push that button' but he could allow me ten minutes beforehand to allow me to say good-bye to her. It was his judgement that she was unlikely to survive the thirty-six hours it would take to get the results of two PCR tests and that I had just ten minutes left. What would you do if you only had ten minutes?

I grabbed my phone and video-called Geoff so that her daddy could tell her how much he loved her, and I could explain to him what was happening. That took about three minutes.

I grabbed a book that I had bought the day before called *The Brave Little Lion* and videoed myself reading it to her as a 'bedtime story' so that they could play it for her if she 'woke up' (if they were able to bring her out of her induced coma) in the isolation room and was scared without me. I also recorded it so they could play it for her if she was going to die and we couldn't be with her, so that she would let go listening to Mummy's voice. That took me up to about five minutes.

I scribbled a quick story about how much her brothers loved her and how much fun they were having with her cousins and Granma.

I held her baby head and I kissed it from her Jelly (this is the name affectionally given to my sister, Jessica, by my children). I told her about how if she went to the other side just to look for the little boy that looked like Campbell because his identical twin and her missing big brother, Benjamin, would be waiting there for her. I told her that if it was too much to keep fighting that I would miss my little shadow and that she was my best friend and that I never regret a single night that she slept in our bed. That her daddy loved her more than any other female in the whole world and that whether she came back or went to the other side she was worth it all and I was so honoured that she chose me to be her mumma.

Around me, nurses were readying the machinery (and a tear or two may have been wiped into their PPE) and they told me I had one more minute. I told her that I would be just outside her room and that her daddy and I would be with her as soon as we could and that as soon as we saw her, we could bake cupcakes and go to the zoo and I'd take her to the dolphin hotel. But that if I couldn't, that this had been enough, and she was enough. And in that moment, I have never loved someone so completely and wholly. In some ways all the trauma that she has experienced across the last few years seemed to have reached a pinnacle, and as they wheeled her away from me and left me in that empty PICU bedspace, I finally let go of something that I'd been holding onto for so long. I let go of the hope that this would ever be over. At what point do you stop asking your child 'be brave, keep fighting' and right there, in that moment, I stopped.

I honestly didn't think I'd ever see her alive again and there was a part of me that was relieved for her. I can't imagine how exhausting it is fighting her big fight and I just couldn't ask her to keep fighting it. So instead, I said goodbye. With a heart full of love and gratitude for the gift she had given me in being my daughter. No matter what happened from here on in I felt a closure on this chapter, and it was closure because I was at peace with it.

That moment of peace I felt (which, to be fair, was really just the shock setting in) was shattered when the security guards arrived to escort me off hospital grounds. When I was told that I couldn't be with Marleigh while she was in isolation, I'd imagined I'd be sitting outside her hospital room, maybe watching her through a glass window? Not realising that as I had been in contact with a potential COVID-19 patient I would be escorted off hospital grounds and not allowed to return until she had been cleared of COVID-19. I will never be the same person that I was before the moment that I understood the reality of our situation. In that moment I finally allowed my heart to succumb to the injustice of it all. My screams and wails of injustice and heartbreak to those I love the most on that day will haunt me forever. Katie, you were the last person who needed to hear it, especially as you understood it all so well and I'll always feel the deepest sense of guilt and gratitude for the space you held for me that day.

In my darkest moments, I can hear echoes of the phone call I made from the hallways of the Sydney Children's Hospital. I sounded like a wounded animal, and I will be forever grateful to my brother Jake for getting me through that day. I don't remember what he said to me, but I do remember the way it made me feel and it helped me to pick myself up off those hospital chairs in the hallway and take the next step.

What we may never recover from is the stories and flashbacks that Marleigh shared with us as she slowly regained her consciousness and ability to communicate. In the weeks to come she would tell us that she, 'Woke up and couldn't find my mummy, so I went outside and up to the rainbow and the rainbow brought me back to my mummy.'

The morning after we said goodbye to Marleigh and she was still in an induced coma, in the PICU isolation room, we woke up the most beautiful double rainbow just after dawn over Coogee Beach. To me, that symbolised that Benjamin had come to let us know that he was taking Marleigh. Having said that, Coogee is also a very special place for Geoff and his family as it is where his father Murray Joseph (whose initials we used to name Marleigh – we've always felt that she was his final gift to us) was living before he passed away the year before Marleigh was born. The day of Murray's funeral, we saw the same double rainbow over Sandy Bay in Hobart, Tasmania. We speak of Murray and Benjamin often, weaving them through our family story and reminding our children that 'just because we can't see them doesn't mean we don't love them, and that they are still a part of our family'. I know that Benjamin has been watching over his sister this whole time and I find it hard to believe that the rainbow story she so enchantedly tells is just a coincidence. But then we have learned that grief is just love. And giving ourselves to embrace that in all its manifestations has been such a such a gift in becoming who we need to be to survive.

Marleigh's final diagnosis was respiratory sepsis, secondary to intubation following her status epilepticus seizure. She tested positive for haemophilus influenzae (HIB), influenza B and streptococcus pneumoniae. None of us tested positive for COVID-19. Everything that happened from 15 May 2020, the status epilepticus seizure, the helicopter, the PICU, the induced coma, ventilator, noradrenaline, security guards ... It was all predicated by Marleigh suffering an acute autoimmune encephalitis relapse, requiring a high dose on IVIG donated by Australian plasma donors.

Geoff and I lay sleepless in a hotel room in Coogee the night we expected her to die, equally willing the phone to ring with news of a negative COVID-19 test but terrified that if it did ring it would be with the news of Marleigh's passing. You would think in a situation like that there is no way that you would leave your child, and I've spent many a night questioning why or how we managed that twenty-nine hours until we were allowed, one by one, to see her again, but I think it's incredibly important to remember the fear surrounding COVID-19 early in the pandemic. I was so acutely aware of the incredible sacrifice that the medical staff were making for my child that morning as they wheeled her away from me. Exposing themselves to my potentially COVID-19-positive child, working tirelessly to save her life, putting their own families at risk by looking after mine.

As we lay awake that night, Geoff and I came up with a plan that if Marleigh survived, we would sell our house in Canberra and everything we owned, move somewhere with a local PICU and warmer weather. Geoff could work from home, and we would soak in every moment that we had with our little family. Not knowing if we would get any more time with Marleigh, or if we did how long that would last.

In September 2023, we just clocked our third anniversary of living on the Sunshine Coast in Queensland, and life in the Fisher family is as hectic as ever, but in the most beautiful way. Marleigh is now in her second year of remission from autoimmune encephalitis and is no longer on a regular IVIG protocol!

She will remain dependent on Australian plasma donors for life due to the risk of relapse, but she is at school part-time, enjoys swimming, dancing and yoga. She's funny, creative, artistic and the most fiercely loyal friend. She can amuse herself for hours with nothing more than a few plastic figurines. It's amazing how the creativity required for amusing yourself in a hospital bed can serve you so well in the years to come! Her autism assistance and seizure response service dog, Paddy, has helped to heal so much of her trauma and bring her so much joy!

Thomas and Campbell absolutely love living on the coast but deeply miss their cousins who are in country New South Wales and I'm not sure that we will ever be forgiven for making them all live apart!

Geoff is still working from home; one of the great blessings of COVID-19 for our family was that when the public service in Canberra sent everyone to work from home for a year or so, we moved to Queensland and Geoff has just kept working from home! The kids are all heartbroken when he has to travel for work for a day or two. They love walking in the front door after school and having him in the front office of our house to share all their stories with. It's meant that rather than travelling to and from work, he has the capacity to volunteer at the school when they need someone to cook a BBQ or help out at events and coach the kids' sports. He is also the audio production manager for the *Milkshakes for Marleigh* podcast and despite the fact that my name is all over it, our blood donation advocacy is a joint pursuit.

I split my time between wrangling our beautiful family with additional needs, running my child-centred play therapy practice part-time, which I set up so that children and their families who had suffered medical trauma could access play therapy outside a hospital setting, and running Milkshakes for Marleigh! Which started as the name of a Lifeblood team people could register their blood donations to and has grown to an entire community of donors and recipients sharing their stories, an award-winning podcast and now this book! All of which are tools in my mission to end persistent critical blood shortages in Australia and around the world. I didn't set out to be a changemaker, but I did develop a creative solution to a social problem, and donors to the Milkshakes for Marleigh Lifeblood team have saved over five thousand lives since I began telling her story, to thank blood donors and encourage new ones.

CHAPTER 12

HUGH VAN CUYLENBURG

Hugh is just the kind of guy that makes you want to strive to be a better person. He describes himself first and foremost and being a dad to children Elsie, Benji and Patrick, husband to Penny, a son and a brother, author, founder of The Resilience Project, creator and co-host of one of Australia's most popular podcasts, *The Imperfects*. Every day, 425,000 Australian students engage with work that he has delivered. He is also a blood donor.

Hugh has been a great supporter of the Milkshakes for Marleigh podcast and I was overwhelmed with gratitude when he agreed to be a guest on my podcast.

Hugh: *'Kate, it's just a nightmare. I couldn't even write a script for a nightmare that's worse than that ... I can't even begin to imagine how brave and resilient Marleigh is ... And one day in the future I hope that you get to sit down with her and explain that all of your work has been inspired by her ... And for her to know how many lives have been saved by you telling her story.'*

When Hugh accepted my invite to be a be a guest on the *Milkshakes for Marleigh* podcast, he wasn't sure that he met the criteria. He told me that he had donated blood but hadn't done it in years and that he'd never needed or loved someone who had needed any type of blood products. While he supported the concept, he didn't think it was really relevant to his life. But when I read his first book, *The Resilience Project*, I found it filled with references to people that Hugh loved who likely needed blood products throughout their lives. I pointed out to him that:

1. 'Beefy' likely needed blood products to address some of his health challenges which have included hydrocephalus, a stroke and cerebral palsy. He features heavily in the book as the team manager for the Melbourne University Cricket Club and has made his mark with his passionate speeches of inspiration and frank and fearless delivery of feedback to players and assessment of the opposition.

2. 'Christie's dad' (Christie was Hugh's first love and first romantic relationship) likely needed blood products during his treatment for blood cancer and/or during his bone marrow transplant.

3. 'Nick Reiwoldt's sister Maddie' (see earlier chapter of this book for the story of Maddie's Vision with Fiona) needed hundreds of blood products during her treatment for bone marrow failure and aplastic anaemia. At the request of Maddie and in her memory, the Reiwoldts continue to be blood donation advocates.

Hugh and I chatted about the misconceptions around who needs blood products. And that most people don't realise that blood isn't just used for major trauma and in a lifesaving capacity, but that it is also used to prolong and improve the quality of people's lives. And in addition, blood donors keep families and loved ones together. I described it as blood donors not just keeping Marleigh alive, but in doing so, also keeping a little sister with her big brothers and a daughter with her parents. A little girl who is insanely loved by her cousins, Jelly, Granma, uncles, aunts and friends. Hugh told me that he had donated blood 'many years ago' and absolutely played it down as not being a big deal. I reminded Hugh that on that day he saved at least three lives. His response: 'See, I just don't think that people know that! I think that if more people knew that giving blood just one time would save three lives, then more people would actually do it!'

And with that, he validated so much of the work I do in my blood donation advocacy and through the *Milkshakes for Marleigh* podcast because if someone like Hugh (who is well-educated and health-conscious, with superior levels of health literacy and has committed his professional life to making the world a better place for his fellow Aussies) doesn't understand the impact and importance of blood donation, then it's reasonable to assume that the majority of Aussies, many of whom are likely less well-resourced than Hugh, who are eligible and able to donate, simply have no idea the impact that a single donation of blood could make, let alone becoming a regular, lifelong blood donor.

Over a year after we released his *Milkshakes for Marleigh* podcast episode, I caught up with Hugh in Brisbane when he was touring *The Imperfects* in a live show format. It was one of the best shows I've ever been to, and to be fair that was supported by the fact that the guest the hosts interviewed was Joe Brum, creator of the Australian children's program, *Bluey* (disclaimer – it's branded as children's entertainment but it's one of my favourite-ever TV shows!). In his discussion with Hugh and his co-hosts, brother Josh van Cuylenberg and comedian Ryan Shelton, Brum explained that his inspiration came from raising his two daughters and wanting to convey the importance of children processing the world around them and understanding their relationship to it through the use of imaginative play. As a child-centred play therapist, I've never nodded so hard along with any interview in my life! And I reflected that the brilliance of *Bluey* isn't just the way that it gives this messaging to children, it's more in the way that it draws in adults to becoming avid followers of the show, and then seeing themselves reflected in the imperfections of Bluey and Bingo's parents, Chilli and Bandit Heeler. That little Aussie family of animated cattle dogs have made me reflect so many times on the importance of encouraging children to build resilience and problem-solving skills, the importance of presence rather than presents, the value of allowing children to be bored and the value of children having periods of time that are unstructured and unscheduled, because this is when they find ways to amuse themselves and this is when they PLAY! As a play therapist, I know that play is important for children because it allows them to make sense of the world around them, establish a sense of identity, increase creativity and reduce impulsive behaviours and aggression while learning to experience and express emotions and finally it cultivates an acknowledgement of the feelings of those around us and supports the development of empathy. I loved the parallels that Joe and Hugh drew between experiences of empathy and vulnerability in the transition to parenthood alongside the authenticity of self in the experience of parenting and how humans learn to parent alongside their offspring who are learning to be human.

Filled with the wonder and raw emotions of *The Imperfects* show, I met Hugh afterwards to give him a gift for being on our podcast. A Milkshakes for Marleigh T-shirt, with a card and gift bag decorated with Marleigh's drawings. Marleigh gave it to him with a simple 'thanks for helping me to get my plasma and being on my podcast' and then was desperate to get back to her daddy and big brothers, who were lurking in the foyer. Such a crowded and high sensory environment isn't great for her autism, functional neurological disorder or brain injury!

Meeting Hugh with Marleigh and having him be so raw and vulnerable on my podcast and so incredibly encouraging and supportive of my work has given me so much drive, and I took Hugh's advice that more people would donate blood if they knew they would save at least three lives and use every opportunity I have to share it with the world.

Hugh speaks of his work with The Resilience Project as the work of his heart, his passion and his soul, and he has impacted the lives of millions of Australians through teaching his gratitude, empathy and mindfulness (GEM) program. He credits his work as being inspired by not wanting another family to have to go through what his family did when his sister Georgia was battling anorexia, which was later discovered to be associated with her experience of childhood sexual assault. I spoke with Hugh about how I see my blood donation advocacy work in the same way and that I never want another family to be scared that there won't be treatment available for their loved one like we were with Marleigh during the critical blood shortages of 2020, when she was on a ten-day treatment cycle and we were never able to look further than ten days ahead, because if she didn't get her next dose of treatment her life was in danger. In the words of her paediatric immunologist:

'For Marleigh, IVIG (intravenous immunoglobulin infusion, made from donated human plasma) is lifesaving when she has an acute relapse and life-preserving for every infusion in-between.'

When he was a guest on my podcast, Hugh and I spoke about Marleigh's experiences of status epilepticus seizures that have lasted up to thirty-nine hours, her time in paediatric intensive care units intubated in an induced coma and the loss of her ability to walk, talk or recognise us as her parents. And as I am so passionate about my mission and Hugh is such a remarkable professional that I respect so deeply, I forgot somewhere in our chat that I was talking to a fellow (sleep-deprived!) parent. And in the end, his empathy got the best of him and he shed tears for our little girl.

Hugh: 'I'm sorry, I just cannot believe everything that your family have gone through ... everything that you have just said is incredibly heartbreaking. As a parent I just don't know how you are doing what you are doing. You (and your husband) are extraordinary ...'

And my response: 'If any of your children needed plasma (or any other blood products) to keep them alive and to keep your family together, you would quit all that you do now and you would make it your life's mission to ensure that enough Australians were donating enough blood so that your child got the treatment they needed.'

I ended our chat by asking Hugh to do me a favour. Next time he and his amazing wife Penny were in the car with their three kids, I wanted him to look at them and realise that statistically at least one of them will be dependent of Australian blood donors to survive, one in three, and yet only about one in thirty eligible donors ever make a blood donation.

I am so grateful to have Hugh as part of the Milkshakes for Marleigh community and supporting my mission to increase the number of blood donors in Australia and reduce the frequent critical blood shortages and by telling these stories, thank as many blood donors as we can along the way.

CHAPTER 13

PHIL DAVIS

In 2023, Phil Davis 'hung up the boots', ending his incredible AFL career, which he finished with the Greater Western Sydney (GWS) Giants. A career that was very nearly cut short, along with his life, when he suffered a kidney laceration when he was tackled during an AFL game in 2014 against the Sydney Swans. Blood donors saved Phil's kidney, his AFL career and his life, and he went on to play for another nine seasons, which included running the GWS Giants onto the field as their captain in the club's first-ever grand final in 2019. Outside the club, Phil is extremely highly regarded as a stellar human and an amazing mate who has made incredible contributions to his community. He has gone on to marry his beautiful wife Greta and if they so choose, one day they may become parents. All moments in time that would not have been possible had people not donated blood in the days before Phil's injury.

When Marleigh first became unwell, Phil Davis was captaining the GWS Giants alongside (now close friend of the Fisher family and one of Marleigh's favourite humans) Callan Ward. The Giants had done a lot of promotional work with the Canberra junior AFL clubs and Marleigh's oldest brother Thomas had been taken in by the allure of all the Giants coming to his under-eights AFL team training nights and giving out free Giants merchandise and so began his passionate support of the Giants.

In 2019, Thomas was chosen as a junior mascot to run alongside the captains and lead the GWS Giants out onto Manuka Oval, Canberra. At the same time, Marleigh had a seizure in the grandstand and was taken to hospital via ambulance. The club followed up with our family to see how Marleigh was recovering and the photo I sent of her in the back of the ambulance in her little GWS Giants jersey found its way around the players, and before we knew it, we had the support of a whole AFL club. Phil made regular video messages and sent them to Thomas and Campbell, checking in on how they were coping with having a sick sister in hospital in Sydney for months at a time while they were in Canberra. Donations to the charity ball that was held for Marleigh to raise money for her seizure response service dog, Paddy. Callan visited Thomas at school and surprised him by knocking on the door of his classroom and taking him out of class to kick a footy, much to the envy of his classmates watching through the windows! Callan visited Marleigh at the Sydney Children's Hospital neurology ward, just after she had been released from the paediatric intensive care unit following an airlift from Canberra, in a critical condition, due to a thirty-nine-hour status epilepticus seizure as a result of autoimmune encephalitis. We came to realise very quickly that while football players get a bit of a bad rap sometimes, these men were some of the most genuine caring humans that we'd ever come across. The majority of these interactions happened off-camera and never found their way to social media. These were not performative acts, they were just the kindness and generosity of spirt shown to our family by an AFL team who had their hearts stolen by a beautiful little girl and the way that her big brothers loved her.

Phil: 'One thing about football and sport is that it can bring people together, and it brought the Fisher family to the Giants. We all hope that we can have happy and healthy lives and when you hear about a child, especially a young child like Marleigh, it touches you ... To think about her in the stands of a game having a seizure, it just really hits home ... We like to see the Giants as a community, and when someone in our community is having a tough time, we do all that we can to help.'

In the years to come and through the Milkshakes for Marleigh blood donation advocacy movement, I learned that like Marleigh, Phil was also a blood product recipient and that he owed his kidney, his AFL career and likely his life to Australian blood donors. In 2014, when playing against the Sydney Swans, twenty-three-year-old Phil was on the end of a standard tackle, just like thousands of tackles before it in his time playing AFL, however, as innocuous as it looked, this caused damage to Phil's kidney that made it 'look like a car crash' when he later went in for surgery. At the time, though, Phil had no idea the extent of his injury. He describes is as a 'moderate knee, moving at a moderate pace, just at the wrong angle at the wrong time'. Immediately, Phil just thought he was winded, or maybe a cracked rib, but he could never have imagined the extent of his injuries. He had no idea that we would be at risk of losing his kidney and that had blood not been available for his initial transfusion and then for the two surgeries, his life would also be in danger.

It wasn't until the morning after the game that Phil understood that something was very wrong. Upon waking, Phil went to the bathroom and instead of passing urine, he passed over 700ml of pure blood. On arrival to the hospital, scans revealed that he had a haematoma the size of a football around his kidney and it appeared to surgeons as 'mush', having split from some of the arteries around it. His first surgery took three hours; his second surgery where he was initially told he would lose his kidney, took a further fourteen hours, during which he would require 'around twenty bags of blood including plasma and platelets transfusions'.

As a twenty-three-year-old, Phil was facing his own mortality head-on for the first time, but his primary concern was that if he lost his kidney, then he would not be able to continue his AFL career.

Phil: 'I am very fortunate that blood was available for me because it bought me the time I needed to have my kidney saved, and that saved my AFL career. Obviously, there were much worse consequences if things didn't go well … this was an area of life I had no understanding of before my injury. You hear about the donating of blood but not in the sense of how it can make a significant difference.'

Following his two weeks in hospital, which included an eight-day stay in an intensive care unit, Phil started the slow process of physical and psychological recovery. One of the big challenges was the massive blood clot that had formed in his abdomen, the other was the psychological aspect of getting back on the field, contesting another football and taking another tackle.

Phil went from running 13km per day to walking a few hundred metres and this being celebrated as an achievement. But he didn't care how long the rehab took, he was deeply committed to leading his GWS Giants back out onto the field.

Phil: 'I remember being asked in the draft process why I wanted to play AFL rather than do something else with my life, and my answer was that I only had this one chance to play AFL while I was young. You can't decide at fifty that you want to give AFL a go, you can only do it while you are young, and when my career is over, the rest of the world will be waiting for me.'

One of the things that drew our attention when Thomas first wanted to start watching GWS Giants' games was the incredible work that the club and players do in the community and the genuine love and respect that they show for each other on the field. One of the reasons that we are so committed to our children playing team sports is so much more than the fitness and fun elements, it's about being part of a team, making a commitment to the other people that will wear the same jersey as you every Saturday morning for a season and showing up for each other every week. It's the closest emulation to what our children will experience in a workplace, and it teaches them things about respect, gratitude and commitment that can only be truly appreciated in a team environment. Off the football field, Phil speaks of his most memorable achievements being the connections that he has made with people.

Phil: 'Some of the most special moments have been the times that we've gone to hospitals and someone can be really sick and it doesn't matter if you see a fifty-year-old or a five-year-old, or someone like Marleigh, if you can make them smile and forget about their illness or their struggles for a few moments, then it's all worthwhile.'

The gift that blood donors give extends past the recipients' lives that are saved, preserved or prolonged and even past the family that love that person. It allows that person to make contributions to their communities that would have otherwise been missed. When Phil retired in August 2023, there was such an amazing amount of commentary about the impact that he has had on the GWS Giants, the AFL as a whole and the community that he has been so committed to building. But I think the words of Phil's close mate and fellow inaugural GWS Giants co-captain, Callan Ward, summed it all up best. His message to Phil was this:

'Wow, what journey … Where do I even start?

'The ultimate teammate – dedicated, trustworthy, loyal, hard-working and courageous. You never left any stone unturned and you got the best out of yourself and everyone around you.

'And one hell of a mate – selfless, positive and ever reliable. You'd do anything to help whenever it was needed, and the love and support that you've shown to me and my family over the years, I'll cherish forever.

'We will all miss you and everything that you bring, and I wish you nothing but success in whatever you choose to do. I love you, mate.'

Thanks to the people who donated the blood that saved his life and his kidney, Phil went on to have an incredible AFL career and captained the GWS Giants at their first grand final in 2019. He's been an incredible mentor, teammate and friend and will be clearly missed at the GWS Giants. He's married to the beautiful Greta, and together they have the chance to make beautiful babies! And as Phil said when he was being drafted, he had his time in the AFL when he was young and 'now the rest of the world is waiting'.

But first, Phil is proud to step into his role as an ambassador for the Milkshakes for Marleigh Lifeblood team and we hope that his fellow Giants will join him in the off-season and become donors for life:

Phil: 'One of the things I look forward to when I retire is becoming a very consistent blood donor. It's such an important part of society and not just for the few people that you help, it gives us all a sense of possibility.'

CHAPTER 14

JESS VAN NOOTEN

Alba is the baby who humanised war for so many Australians who couldn't fathom the atrocities of war. When Russia invaded Ukraine on 24 February 2022, Aussies watched news reports about a country that felt so far from our own. Within days, our social media and news feeds were flooded with stories of Aussies impacted by the conflict, but one story struck hearts in a particular way. The story of an Australian baby fighting for her life in the middle of the conflict. She had been born prematurely via her surrogate in a Ukrainian hospital just hours before Russia invaded, and her parents Kev and Jess were in a desperate attempt to retrieve their baby girl from the conflict zone in Ukraine and #bringalbahome to Australia.

Jess: 'If the Ukrainian people hadn't donated the blood Alba needed in the days before she was born, she wouldn't have survived ... and the people that donated the blood she needed in London ... and the thousands of Australians who have donated the blood that Marleigh needs ... We are just two mums dependent on blood donors from all over the world to keep our daughters alive.'

Chefs Kev and Jess have been together for twenty-two years. They met, fell in love, travelled the world and then settled down to have a family. They wanted to have a baby and thought, *It can't be that hard?* But they quickly found that the contraceptives they had been using for so many years likely weren't needed, as an autoimmune condition was preventing Jess from sustaining pregnancies. After a long, long in-vitro fertilisation (IVF) journey, including fourteen embryo transfers, some that resulted in pregnancies, some that resulted in miscarriage, but none that resulted in a baby in Jess and Kev's arms and seven years of primary infertility, they decided that they needed to try something different.

Jess: 'IVF is a roller-coaster! It is an awesome thing if it works, but if it doesn't you are on the bottom of that roller-coaster for a very long time.'

Jess and Kev decided to pursue the option of surrogacy. After much research they picked a surrogacy agency in Ukraine. With the use of Jess' eggs and Kev's sperm, embryos were created in Australia and then transported to Ukraine to be transferred into the surrogate that they had selected, with support from the surrogacy agency. Due to the COVID-19 pandemic, they met their Russian-speaking surrogate via video call, and with the use of a translator, they knew that this surrogate was the one. The main hurdle (among all the other obvious complications!) they came up against is that Jess and Kev weren't married – having poured all their financial, emotional and physical resources into fifteen rounds of IVF in the last seven years, it just hadn't been at the top of the priority list. But this was a requirement to access a surrogate in Ukraine. With a small group of family and friends present, they tied the knot so that they could ship their five frozen embryos to Ukraine. They chose the 'strongest' of the five embryos (who would go on to be baby Alba) to be transferred into the Ukrainian surrogate.

Anyone who has experienced IVF knows the dreaded two-week wait following an embryo transfer where you wait to see if it has resulted in pregnancy. Having your embryo in a surrogate in Ukraine and waiting for a text message to see if it had worked was excruciating for Jess, who described herself as a 'bit of a control freak!'. But in the middle of the night the text message lit up her phone screen and a delighted Jess woke Kev to tell him, 'We are pregnant!' As Alba was a genetically tested embryo, their Australian-based fertility clinic had all her information and as soon as the pregnancy reached twelve weeks, Kevin and Jess were able to access those details and found out that she was a girl! And only then could Jess set foot in a baby store – given their experience of recurrent pregnancy loss they had a hard time believing it was real.

The plan was for Jess and her mumto leave Australia to fly to Ukraine on 25 April 2022 and settle into the seaside town two weeks ahead of Alba's due date of 11 May 2022. Alba's daddy, Kev, would come straight over as soon as she was born. The strict COVID-19 protocols dictated that even though she was genetically theirs, Jess and Kev were not able to meet baby Alba until she was four days old. But that plan dramatically changed.

At twenty-eight weeks and four days into the pregnancy, Jess received a message informing her that Alba's surrogate had been hospitalised with a sore back. She reported that she was not too alarmed as she knew how well Ukrainian surrogates were looked after and that twelve weeks into the pregnancy, the surrogate had been put on bed rest in hospital for two weeks due to an irritable uterus. The next message that Jess received, while Kev was at work and she was home alone, read:

Hello. Your baby has been born unexpectedly. She is alive, for the moment.

Jess describes the next twenty-four hours as a blur. The only way that she could get information was through the Ukrainian surrogacy agency. She couldn't speak Russian and she couldn't even call the hospital to check on her baby and she didn't even know which hospital she was in. But she did know that she was a mother and her baby needed her, so she and Kev got on the first flight they could to get to their baby girl.

Jess: 'We got a call from the Australian government asking us not to travel to Ukraine, but we didn't even consider it. We needed to get to Alba.'

On reflection, Jess now knows that the survival of her premature baby girl hinged on how many people had donated blood in the city of Odessa in the days before Alba was born, because without these transfusions she would not be able to survive. Blood donation would not be at the top of the priority list for the citizens of the Ukraine in the days to follow, as while Jess' flight was in the air, Russia invaded Ukraine.

Jess describes landing in Dubai for a stop-over on her way from Australia to Ukraine and turning her phone on, desperate for news about whether their baby girl was still alive. They ordered a bottle of champagne, so excited that in four hours they were getting on the plane to FINALLY meet their baby. And then

Jess' phone rang again, and the Australian government updated them on Russia invading Ukraine and explained that all flights had been cancelled and they would not be travelling to Odessa to meet their baby.

The updates that Jess and Kev received in the next few weeks while they tried desperately to get to their baby girl were terrifying. Jess describes how she never conceptualised that Alba would be sick, she just thought she was born really small and needed to grow bigger so that she could come home! One of the first proper updates they got was terrifying:

Jess: 'We received a video message when we arrived at the hotel in Warsaw, it had been translated from Russian and it told us that Alba had a severe bleed on both sides of her brain, underdeveloped lungs and an underdeveloped intestinal system. We didn't know what any of that meant and we didn't get another update for two days. But we didn't speak Russian and the hospital was in the middle of a warzone, it was impossible for us to contact anyone.'

Jess and Kev went on to learn that the life of their surrogate, who they affectionately refer to as 'Alba's tummy mummy', was also saved by blood donors as she suffered a life-threatening postpartum haemorrhage and required a blood transfusion. When she was discharged from hospital following Alba's birth, she was unable to get to her husband and two children, due to the conflict that surrounded her, so instead she offered her time volunteering to help other mothers and their children at the hospital, some of whom were also displaced by the war.

Jess describes finally meeting Alba as surreal. When she and Kev arrived at the hospital, they were surprised to see dogs roaming freely around, and when they washed their hands they used a communal cloth hand towel, a far cry for the hygiene and sanitisation procedures in place at neonatal intensive care units in Australian hospitals. They were led down hallways peering into rooms and wondering which one was their baby. And when they finally met her, rather than the overwhelming joy and love they had dreamed of, it was a feeling of worry and fear. Alba looked very small and very unwell.

One of the great challenges that they faced was the language barrier. Nobody told them if they could touch their daughter, nobody had referred to her as 'Alba' before Kev and Jess arrived, nobody could give them updates. But what they knew was that Alba wasn't safe with the conflict coming closer to the hospital and they weren't sure that she was getting the best medical treatment possible. An example is that Alba had a brain surgery conducted while she was still in her bed, plastic bags full of surgical equipment were emptied on her bedside to complete the procedure. When Jess arrived at the hospital a few days later, she found a dirty stuffed toy sitting on Alba's head, in contact with where she'd had her surgery. These are the memories that hit her when she tells the story of knowing they needed to get her out of Ukraine.

Kev and Jess were met with opposition from the hospital staff in Ukraine, and through the language barrier, they argued. What became clear was that there was risk in transporting Alba when she was so unwell. But there was also great risk in not moving her to a better-resourced hospital that was not in the middle of a warzone. The doctors told Jess: 'If you leave and she dies, it's your fault.'

But Jess trusted her mumma gut, and via Moldova they finally got her out of Ukraine and to the Great Ormond Street Hospital in London where they spent the next four months. Among the many challenges that Alba faced while there, one of them was that Kev and Jess, although her biological parents and named on her birth certificate, were not recognised as her legal guardians, which made it super tricky for them to give consent for her multiple blood transfusions and brain surgery. They themselves were not even able to donate blood while they were there as it was during the COVID-19 pandemic, and their international travel disqualified them as donors.

In the end, Jess and Kev did get to #bringalbahome to Australia, and today, thanks to blood donors across the globe, Alba lives a beautiful big life! Jess is working in the kitchen at the child care centre she attends so is 'never more than 10m away from Alba'. Alba had additional challenges associated with her premature arrival and the medical events that followed including cerebral palsy, infantile spasms and developmental delays. She has a regular schedule of medical and therapy appointments and will always be impacted by her early arrival. However, her survival is nothing short of astonishing, and Kev, Jess and Alba adore being a family and the simple pleasures that it brings. Something that they longed for for such a long time and will never take for granted.

Jess: 'We are so overwhelmed by the kindness and messages from people all over the world, the financial contributions and the blood donors from Ukraine and the United Kingdom who saved Alba's life and the life of our surrogate. We know that people donated blood in Australia for her too and it means so much to us as a family.'

Alba's story humanised war for so many Australians, who through acts of patriotism, love and virtue signalling, made the hashtag #bringalbahome go viral. This helped in the exposure of Jess and Kev's fundraising campaign, organised by their loved ones, to ensure that they had the financial resources to retrieve their baby girl. However, I can't help but wonder if Alba had been born in Australia and needed blood products, would the same people have donated blood to ensure her survival?

I am so grateful to Jess for so candidly sharing her journey of infertility, pregnancy loss and surrogacy with me. That alone is an epic journey, without the complication having to get your premmie fragile baby out of a warzone.

Jess is a blood and plasma donor; she encourages those in her network to donate as well. When we spoke, she was organising a group of people from her workplace to donate blood and she told me about her sister who has made over one hundred plasma donations. Together, we reflected on how blood donors don't just save lives, they keep families together. And how grateful we are that blood donors from all over the world have kept Alba and Marleigh with us, their mummas.

CHAPTER 15

CHRIS BOND

Chris Bond is a two-time world champion wheelchair rugby player. He has competed at three summer Paralympics and was a gold medallist at the 2012 London and 2016 Rio Paralympics. In 2022, he captained Australia to winning the wheelchair rugby world championships. He is married to fellow para-athlete, Dr Bridie Kean who is an Australian wheelchair basketball player. She won a bronze medal at the 2008 Beijing Paralympics and a silver medal at the 2012 London Paralympics. Together they have three children, two of them are living. They are raising their family together on the Sunshine Coast in Queensland, while making incredible contributions to their professional and sporting lives and making the world a better place for others through their volunteer work and contributions to their communities. None of this would be possible without the generosity of Australian blood donors.

Chris: 'I was always known as the sporty kid. Always going to state championships for different sports ... afternoons after school were always riding bikes or pulling up wheelie bins in the street to play cricket. I've always been really active, it's just been my life ... And there was that one defining moment in hospital when the doctor came in an explained what my amputations would be by drawing a stick figure and showing me what they were taking off. That was the moment that reality set in for me.'

Chris was a carefree nineteen-year-old working in hospitality and enjoying weekends at the pubs around Canberra when his life took a very dramatic turn. He started feeling unwell and experiencing some abdominal pain, initially he thought this may be a gastro virus or food poisoning.

Chris: 'I was fit, healthy, in shape. I was always up for a few drinks with mates on a weekend and getting up to some mischief you probably wouldn't tell your mother about but nothing more than a bit of occasional binge drinking. I was working towards a career in the hospitality industry. But then I noticed I was feeling a bit run down, nothing terrible because I was in pretty good shape.'

Chris went to the doctor and was prescribed antibiotics for a suspected infection. He says in hindsight he also had some bleeding of his gums, but nothing that concerned him too much. He had a few weeks off work to rest but then wanted to get back into it. He went to work, worked the first half of his shift at the restaurant despite the fatigue he was feeling but when break time came, he wasn't hungry and couldn't eat. This concerned his bosses, who were used to seeing the appetite of an active nineteen-year-old, enough that they send him home to rest, with the intention of him returning the next day. Over the next twenty-four hours, Chris experienced stabbing abdominal pain, followed by diarrhoea and vomiting. He went to his GP who sent him to the hospital with suspected appendicitis. By this point, Chris was unable to walk and describes crawling across the floor and vomiting uncontrollably. On arrival at the hospital, he was taken straight in for some testing and the results shocked everyone.

Chris: 'I was rushed into emergency, the doctors took me in and did some tests, and the next thing I knew, they said, "We have to take you straight in for an operation and you need to say goodbye to your family, your body is shutting down and we don't like your chances of survival," it was literally that quick. I got the chance to ring my mum and then I rang my best mate and just said, "Thanks for being there," which was a super weird thing to have to do at nineteen. Mum arrived as I was being taken to theatre and all I could do was wave, it all just happened so quickly. And against the odds they had given me, I woke up in a hospital room three days later … induced coma, tubes down my throat, my body was dark purple and black and thinking, *What has happened?* I was on life support, and I saw the doctors put their heads down every time they walked past, they didn't think I was going to survive. That's a reflection of how acute my illness was.'

Once Chris could communicate, all he wanted to know was 'what the hell happened?' it was explained to him that he had a blood cancer called acute promyelocytic leukaemia (APML), which was the cause of the original fatigue and had stripped Chris of his immune system. Chris had also developed the bacterial infection necrotising fasciitis. This is better known as 'flesh-eating disease', and results in the progressive death of soft tissue in the human body. Chris isn't sure where he could have come into contact with the bacteria, but he says: 'As a very active kid, I could have come into contact with it in the bush? A storm water drain? A creek? Who knows, I was always out and about doing something. The APML and the necrotising fasciitis weren't related, just two unfortunate events that happened at the same time. I'd probably had the cancer for a while, but I was young, fit and healthy so just pushing through. One or the other of these things is pretty bad but having them together meant that my body didn't have the immune system to fight an infection, so it just started shutting down.'

Chris' body was so swollen that they had to keep cutting him open to relieve the pressure. He was being given constant intra-venous antibiotics and blood transfusions in an attempt to flush the infection out of his body. During one of his surgeries, his body went into septic shock while he was on the operating table, and it just started shutting down his extremities in an attempt to continue the blood flow to his vital organs. Chris went into cardiac arrest multiple times, dying a few times and requiring defibrillators to shock him back to life. He was then placed into induced coma and was given very little chance of survival.

Against all odds, Chris did survive, and he spent the next month in an intensive care unit (ICU) while his body recov-ered. His kidneys had shut down, requiring dialysis. The sepsis resulted in his body stopping blood supply to his limbs and they died during this time. There was also nothing that could be done about his APML as his body would not have been able to tolerate the treatment.

Chris: 'It took a while for it all to sink in, and even then,

I didn't understand what any of it meant. I didn't know what cancer was. I'd never even been to hospital before this except for a broken wrist, so it was all sinking in and then it all hit me that this was my new life, and it was so hard to see past this when my whole life had been so active and then seeing your body parts die off and thinking I'd never be able to do anything with my life.'

Once he was stable enough to leave the ICU, the next move for Chris was to the infectious diseases ward for another ten months where they could address the necrotising fasciitis and 'all the other infections I'd picked up in hospital like golden staph and MRSA while having open wounds', and only then was Chris stable enough to begin chemotherapy treatment for his cancer.

Chris describes these ten months in flashes of horror that I struggle to even imagine, including daily debridements of the skin from his body, where a scalpel would be used every day to cut away any skin that had died and then his body would be rebandaged to see what would survive and what would die overnight, and Chris says that is about as painful and horrific as it sounds.

Chris: 'Then one day the doctor comes in and says that he knows where the infection is and what can be saved. He told me that they were going to take my left hand and most of my right fingers first and then give it a couple of weeks and then they were going to amputate both of my legs below the knee. That was the moment that reality set in. I felt like my life was over.'

Chris describes the mental and physical health aspects as having equal impact. He was entirely debilitated and traumatised by going from the 'good-looking, sporty kid' to feeling 'like a baby again'. He describes feeling embarrassed and emasculated by the daily sponge baths and being spoon-fed. His mother later told him that in those early months he had sobbed and begged her to 'unplug him' to end the pain and humiliation. His ultimate frustration was that because he was so debilitated, he couldn't even end his own life. He speaks of the old cliché, that 'time heals all', as being so true for him in his physical and mental health recovery.

Chris largely skips past the months and years of cancer treatment and rehabilitation when telling his own story but knows that returning to sport was key to him living a fulfilling life and setting goals for the future. He started completing parts of his physical rehabilitation program at one of the gyms at the Australian Institute of Sport (AIS) and watched on as world-class athletes trained around him, then he started asking questions about becoming a para-athlete and what sports he would be able to be competitive in with his disability. The first suggestion was swimming, and while sceptical as he had been a runner all his life, he decided to give it a crack, but he wasn't so into the 5am frosty starts in a Canberra winter to follow the black line on the bottom on the pool, and he was desperately missing team sports.

In a chance meeting, the Australian wheelchair rugby team were in the gym at the AIS at the same time as Chris one day and his first thought was, *Sign me up!* He'd never seen wheelchair rugby played but was interested! He learned that it's a full-contact team sport, played by both men and women on the same team.

Chris: 'It's like a mix of American sports like gridiron, ice hockey, basketball and a bit of soccer. In terms of stopping people, that's why they called it rugby, it's full-contact and people do get tipped over. The best way to describe it is like dodgem cars mixed with chess, hitting anyone as hard as you like but very strategic once you get to the highest levels. And there is a diverse level of impairments on any team, so it's incredibly tactical and a lot of fun.'

Chris' love for the sport grew quickly and has now seen him represent Australia at three Paralympic games, bringing home gold medals from two. Among his many sporting achievements as a para-athlete, captaining the Australian wheelchair rugby team to winning the 2022 World Cup seems to stand out for him. Maybe because it came at such a difficult time in his family's life, just months after the birth of their twin sons.

Chris speaks with so much pride when he talks about his wife Bridie and the family that they are raising together. He shares the incredible work that she has done on Australia's bid for the Brisbane 2032 Olympic and Paralympic Games and her commitment to using it as an opportunity to ensure that Australia is recognised as a leader in accessible tourism. More recently, Chris and Bridie presented together at the Gender Equality Symposium, an event that ran alongside the 2023 FIFA Women's World Cup, where they presented to over two hundred world leaders, academics, athletes and advocates about the importance of gender equality in sport and the benefits this has to broader communities. When you tally these incredible personal and professional achievements, Paralympic medals, volunteer work and contributions to their communities, it's such a clear illustration of the gift that blood donors give when they save, prolong or improve the quality of people's lives as they did for Bridie when she had a life-threatening meningococcal infection that resulted in the amputation of her legs and Chris' APML and sepsis, which left him a quad-amputee.

Not only have Chris and Bridie survived these illnesses, but they have gone on to create more lives! Chris and Bridie welcomed their first child in 2019 and then their twins in 2022. They are raising two of these children on the beautiful Sunshine Coast, while remembering baby Alexander.

Chris: 'Bridie and I lost a child. One of our twins died, and so I know about acute fear and grief now. It's given me a very different insight into how my illness affected my parents, siblings, friends and loved ones. It adds a new layer to how much I admire my mum and everything she did during my illness.

'We knew early on in the pregnancy that there was a problem with swelling on his brain and we had to make decisions about whether to terminate and what risk that would pose to his twin brother … But he was born and passed away in my arms twenty minutes after. He took his final breath in my arms. It's very raw and very confronting. My partner is a survivor of meningococcal and a double amputee, I'm a quadruple amputee, and our resilience has helped us to take on a challenge like this, not that it makes it any easier, but we have coping skills and we know that's life, I guess. It's a weird silver lining, we lost one son, but we've got one too, it's not all sad, there are some joys as well.'

For now, Chris has his sights set on the 2024 Paris Paralympics, and while he thinks these will be his last, he is really excited to be part of the culture that continues to build on the successes of wheelchair rugby and para-athletes in the future. He is passionate about advocating, alongside Bridie, for improved accessibility in public spaces in Australia for people of all abilities. And he is very excited about his retirement from international sport in the future, meaning that he has more time to be at home with his kids and enjoy being a dad and taking them to all their sports. He knows that none of this would be possible without Australian blood donors.

His message to those blood donors who made the sixty operations, skin grafts, bone marrow transplants, chemotherapy and recovery from sepsis possible:

Chris: 'Thank you! Just thank you! My dad has always been a blood donor, he's a massive advocate for blood donation and has given over one hundred times in his life. Maybe I have had his blood, who knows? So please just donate, I wish I could!'

CHAPTER 16

HUNTER VALLEY BUS TRAGEDY

Duane Roy was chairman of the Maitland Saints Australian Football League (AFL) Club, when the horrific Hunter Valley bus tragedy occurred. With so many people in his local community affected, he knew that he needed to do something to alleviate the sense of hopelessness in the face of this tragedy. Duane coordinated the overwhelming community response in registering new blood donors and their lifelong commitments to blood donation, to honour the memory and celebrate the lives of the bus crash victims.

Duane: 'I must admit I've been taken aback by the generosity of our community to donate blood without really understanding what their blood will do, but just wanting to help. I'm hoping that this will be something that we can focus on long-term.'

On 11 June 2023, a bus transferring the wedding guests of Mitchell Gaffney and Maddy Edsell at Wandin Valley Estate overturned at a roundabout in the country town of Greta in the

New South Wales Hunter Valley. The accident left ten passengers dead and another twenty-five in hospital. A scene of unimaginable horror awaited emergency services as they attended this accident, as with many tight-knit communities, those responding were familiar with some of those on that bus. This was a story that dominated news headlines in Australia and all over the world at the time of the accident and has continued to do so as the surviving driver of the bus, a fifty-eight-year-old man named Brett Button, was charged with dangerous driving occasioning death – drive manner dangerous and negligent driving occasioning death. At the time of printing this book, the case was not yet finalised.

As the local community and its surrounds came to terms with the unspeakable tragedy, local groups, and particularly AFL clubs, put out a call to recruit blood donors to ensure enough blood was available to treat the injuries, infections and burns of the survivors and ensure their safety during the many surgeries they had ahead. Furthermore, donors committed to a lifetime of regular donations as a way to remember those who had died in this horrific accident and in the hope of preventing some of that pain and grief they were experiencing by saving the lives of three fellow Aussies for each blood donation made.

The rally for blood donations captured the attention of small-town local clubs all the way through to the professional AFL clubs. Many of the guests on the bus were members or loved ones of the Singleton Roosters AFL Club and some played at a representative level, having connections to the Sydney Swans Academy Program. The Sydney Swans and many other AFL clubs wore black arm bands the following weekend to remember those who lost their lives. The AFL have also become active participants in blood donation advocacy and rivalries have commenced between club members and supporters to see who can donate the most blood each year. Duane Roy spoke to me about what this recognition means to those affected and the gravity of the grief that has shaken the collection of small communities around Singleton and the Hunter Valley of NSW.

Duane: 'When you have a connection to something like this and a like-minded community, there is a sense of hopelessness when there is just nothing that you can do. We put our heads together and thought that donating blood was something that we could do for the people affected in this tragedy and also to pay it forward, especially when we understood just how much blood was needed following the tragedy in Greta.'

When tragedies of this magnitude occur, people are often told to 'look for the helpers', as this grounds us back to the good in the world, reduces the terror of the onlooker and restores faith in humanity. The difficulty of applying this notion to a tragedy that requires lifesaving blood in acute settings is that the recipients are at the mercy of whether enough blood had been donated in the lead-up to this emergency to fulfil the massive orders placed by John Hunter Hospital, where most of the patients were transferred. At 1am on the morning of Monday 12 June 2023, Lifeblood received a massive order of blood to sustain the lives of those who had been injured and to allow for surgery, treatment of burns and infections of the survivors in the coming days. Within forty minutes of the request, Lifeblood dispatched twenty shippers with 150 units of red cells, plasma and platelets. That was what the hospital needed just for the first night.

Survivors needed ongoing treatment and surgery requiring

blood in the days and weeks to come, and that need was serviced by the blood donations of the people of the Hunter Valley and surrounds. The first season of the *Milkshakes for Marleigh* podcast explored the suggestion that: 'Nothing feels more Australian, like the modern demonstration of "mateship", than donating blood and this being used to keep another Australian alive.'

Nothing shall ever relieve the grief of this senseless tragedy, but the people of the Hunter Valley and surrounds, through their blood donation drive, demonstrated a very productive and generous way to relieve their sense of hopelessness in the face of this heartbreaking tragedy. May those who lost their lives, rest in peace. And those left behind continue to be supported by their communities now and into the future.

CHAPTER 17

ADEM CROSBY

Adem Crosby was many things. He was well-liked, kind, funny, a loyal friend and a lover of music. He played guitar in a band, he was popular with the girls, hardworking and extremely close to his siblings. He was also dying from leukaemia. He captured the hearts of those on the Sunshine Coast, Queensland, who saw his brave fight as a young man who should have been planning to travel, study, map a career, fall in love or start a family. Yet, instead, he had to plan the way that he wanted to die. Following his passing in 2013 at just nineteen years old, his mother Lu and father Brent have continued their blood donation advocacy and commitment to making the lives of families who have children with cancer just a little bit easier.

Lu: '*The giant headline on the front page of the paper read* Local boy Adem loses battle, *but he didn't lose any battle. Our boy was a winner and his legacy lives on.*'

Brent: '*We have so many incredible supporters, without them there would be no Team Adem community or blood donation team.*

It was something that Adem was very passionate about, and we learned very quickly how important those blood products are.'

The courage in Adem's fight and the love that his supporters have for him and the Crosby family is reflected every day by the people who donate blood for the Team Adem Lifeblood team. When you make a blood donation in Australia, you can attribute it to a particular 'team'. These are often formed by organisations as part of blood donor challenges, for example the Commonwealth Government departments in Canberra have a challenge every year to see who can generate the greatest number of donors, or teams can be formed in support of a particular person or cause. The Milkshakes for Marleigh Lifeblood team was formed in 2020 when Marleigh was at her sickest and reliant on intravenous immunoglobulin infusions (IVIG), which is made from donated human plasma, to stay alive. This was also during the COVID-19 pandemic amidst persistent critical blood shortages. The Milkshakes for Marleigh Lifeblood team is incredibly proud to have saved the lives of over five thousand Aussies since 2020. The Team Adem Lifeblood team has saved the lives of nearly 150,000 people since 2013. This number is reflective of the immense impact that Adem had on this world in a life that was way too short and the incredible work that his parents, Brent and Lu, and their supporters continue to do to celebrate his legacy.

Adem Crosby was living the life of a typical Aussie teenager. He was working part-time at a local IGA supermarket and loved listening to music and spending time with friends. He was two days into year twelve, his final year of school, and was excited to be taking on a role as a school prefect. Adem had been experiencing some persistent fatigue and general malaise. His mum Lu had taken him to the doctor just before he started his final year of school and requested blood tests as she knew something wasn't quite right with her boy. But it was brushed off as 'helicopter parenting' and the GP was more worried about Lu overparenting her sixteen-year-old son rather than Adem's physical health.

Two weeks later, the fatigue hadn't resolved, and Adem had started having night sweats and had developed a rash that his parents now recognise at petechiae – which develops from low platelets. Adem came home from his first day of year twelve after spending the day in his role as school prefect and ambassador, welcoming new students to the school, and complained of feeling tired and run down. The next day he collapsed at work while completing his afterschool shift at the local IGA supermarket, and it was very clear that Lu's motherly intuition was absolutely right, and something was very wrong with her son. She took him to a different doctor who sought testing and received a phone call the same night asking the Crosbys to come in for an appointment at 8am the next morning. During this appointment, just five days after his seventeenth birthday, Adem would be informed that he had acute leukaemia and the Crosbys' lives would never look the same again.

Brent: 'His appointment was at 8am, and they told us of the diagnosis of acute leukaemia. By noon he'd already been admitted to the Royal Brisbane Hospital and started receiving treatment, still wearing his school uniform. From that day on our lives changed. We thought we might be there for a week or two but that's where we spent the next two years.'

Adem's siblings had gone to school that morning unconcerned about the doctor's appointment their brother had gone
to. The family thought it may just be a virus, or at worst he might
need an iron infusion. But they were collected from school by
grandparents, and at the insistence of Adem's doctors, rushed
down to Brisbane to see their gravely ill brother, who had spent
the day receiving blood transfusions after arriving at hospital
with a platelet count of just twelve. (The normal platelet count
range for a healthy adult is between 150,000 and 400,000 per
microlitre.)

Lu: 'The doctors wanted Adem's siblings to be with him
because he was just so unwell, and they didn't know what tomorrow would bring. So, we were all together for those early times.
But as he was receiving blood – thank goodness for the gift of
blood – he started feeling better straightaway, and then he had
to get right into treatment. And it was very harsh treatment.'

Initially, Brent, Lu, Adem and his siblings all relocated to
Brisbane. His siblings attended the Royal Brisbane Hospital
School but when it was evident this was not going to be a short
stay in Brisbane, the Crosbys needed to make some big choices.
Brent left his job and stayed in Brisbane full-time with Adem,
with Lu returning to the Sunshine Coast with Adem's younger
siblings and visiting every weekend.

Adem spent twelve months in Brisbane having treatment.
The first six months as an inpatient and the second six months
outpatient, during which time the Crosbys were able to access
accommodation through the Leukaemia Foundation. It was this
accommodation that started them on their advocacy and fundraising journey. First, it was raising money for the Leukaemia

Foundation where Lu shaved her head for 'Team Adem' in the World's Greatest Shave. But Adem wanted to do more, not for himself, but for the others like him that were battling cancer.

Brent: 'He didn't want money for himself, he said, "What I want is to raise money to help all of the other people like me. Look at all those people staying at the Leukaemia Foundation accommodation, let's help them! Let's try to raise money to find a cure! I've got all I need – a family who love me and access to all the treatment I need. Let's help all the others." So guided by Adem, that's what we did.'

Adem survived that first year of treatment and returned to the Sunshine Coast to complete his studies. While he required constant monitoring, the Crosbys wanted to put the nightmare behind them and get on with their lives. Adem had set the goal of becoming an oncology nurse, on the promise of the Royal Brisbane Hospital when he got through that first year of treatment and completed his education that they would have a job waiting for him. During that year he was in remission, Adem was a fierce blood donation advocate, speaking to media and at many events on the importance of blood donation for people with cancer.

Adem completed high school and was accepted into university to complete his studies. As they celebrated one year of remission, Brent and Lu went back to work and tried to move on with their lives, wanting to close the cancer chapter. But unfortunately, this snapshot of normality was very short-lived. Adem was in his first week of university when he was diagnosed with an acute leukaemia relapse. The Crosbys knew that a relapse post-bone marrow transplant was going to be extraordinarily difficult to treat. But Adem wanted to keep trying, and with the help of so many blood transfusions, he kept fighting and underwent so many gruelling treatments in a bid to stay alive. On Lu's fiftieth birthday, Adem had a conversation that would once again change their lives forever.

Brent: 'I remember when the consultant called us in and he just said, "Adem, we have run out of options," and it was incredible, Adem just stood up and hugged him and said, "I thank you so much for everything that you have done for me. I have won this battle. I've done every treatment and everything that's been asked of me. I didn't lose this battle," and when we walked out, I saw that the consultant was crying.'

Adem surprised everyone with his acceptance of running out of treatment options and knowing that he was going to die. He used this time to set up the fundraising and advocacy projects that would become his legacy through Team Adem, all centred around encouraging people to donate blood and making the lives of cancer families easier.

The Crosbys held six consecutive World's Greatest Shave events, raising over $660,000 for the Leukaemia Foundation, all because Adem wanted to help others in need. At the last of these events in 2013, Adem told his supporters that it would be his last. Despite being extremely unwell, he wanted to make one final public appearance to thank his supporters and encourage them to continue his legacy. Adem died six weeks after that event.

Brent: 'We know that a single blood donation can save three lives, but we don't talk enough about blood products helping to *prolong* so many lives. Even those patients who aren't going to have the outcomes that they want, those blood products can give them time to create special memories that will be so special to their loved ones for the rest of their lives.'

When Adem was a little boy, Lu recounts him describing everything as 'so good!' and she knows how proud he would be of the Team Adem blood donation community, and the impact of his story keeps growing. In 2013 he was posthumously awarded the Young Queensland Philanthropy Award, which was accepted on his behalf by his thirteen-year-old brother. The Sunshine Coast University Hospital named their cancer treatment centre 'The Adem Crosby Cancer Centre' to recognise his incredible contributions.

Unfortunately, cancer in the Crosby family didn't end with Adem. Two years after his passing, Lu was diagnosed with breast cancer and was devastated when chemotherapy stopped her from being able to donate blood. A common misconception is that if you've had cancer, you can never donate again, but once she was five years free of cancer and with the clearance of her doctors, she has been able to make regular blood donations to Team Adem again.

Lu: 'It really messed me up for a while, because I thought maybe the reason that this has happened is so that I can die and be with my son. But all bereaved mothers feel like that and it is not really that they want to be with their children, it's that they want their children to be back with them … and I looked into the eyes of my living children and knew that I still needed to be here. What was hard was that I was treated in the same hospital that Adem was born and died in. His photo is on the wall every-where … I just had to compartmentalise.'

Brent and Lu reflect that they think that Adem set them up

with so many projects to complete in his legacy because he knew that they would need them to be able to survive losing him. His last words to Brent before he passed away were around looking after his mum and keeping her strong. Even in his final moments, his thoughts were not of himself, but of those around him.

Lu: 'How did we, ordinary people, working hard and raising a young family in Buderim ... How did this amazing boy come to us? We only had him for a short time, but he's left such an amazing impact on his community and abroad ... He supported so many people in that hospital, he supported us.'

Team Adem is more than a Lifeblood team and blood donation advocacy movement; it has extended to be an incredible charity that makes a profound impact on children and their families who are affected by childhood cancer. The legacy of Team Adem continues to spread love, support and kindness, and Brent and Lu hold role of bereaved parents and carers with such fierce ongoing love for their son and a commitment to making the lives of families battling childhood cancer just a little bit easier.

Lu: 'Adem received over 350 blood products and transfusions during his treatment. We are just so grateful to all the blood donors who made that possible. It gave us more time.

'Adem was the one behind the blood donation advocacy, we wanted to encourage his friends and his community to roll up their sleeves, not just for him, but to help others as well.'

CHAPTER 18

MANDY McCRACKEN

In 2013, Mandy McCracken and her husband Rod were working hard and raising their young family when she became unwell with what she thought was the flu. Within days she would be in an intensive care unit (ICU) fighting for her life from the sepsis that would progressively attempt to destroy her body. Mandy survived with thanks to Australian blood donors and now shares her experiences to help fellow quad-amputees and other people living with disability.

Mandy: 'They had to do the amputations to keep me alive, but I was able to keep my elbow and knee joints. This means that I can use prosthetic legs to walk, and my elbows mean that I can use hooks for hands. I don't even notice the prosthetics anymore, I just crack on, I've got things to do! When you've had your hands and feet chopped off you can pretty much deal with anything.'

At the age of thirty-nine, Mandy McCracken was raising her three young daughters, aged nine, seven and four, alongside husband Rod when she started to feel a little bit unwell. Juggling the mental load of motherhood, children's activities, volunteering and school committees, Mandy was used to feeling tired, but this felt more like a virus, she thought maybe she was coming down with influenza or gastro. It was a Wednesday night and Mandy went to bed early, in the hope she could sleep off whatever was making her feel unwell and then get on with the rest of her week. There was no indication that by that Friday night she would be in an intensive care unit fighting for her life.

Mandy: 'I had a thing called sepsis, which I'd never heard of. It's a reaction to an infection, it's a medical emergency. Your body shuts down and attacks itself. Your body tries to keep your internal organs going so it shuts down circulation. So, my hands and feet eventually turned black, and I ended up with four amputations.'

Mandy speaks of the ten days she was in an induced coma as being 'overall enjoyable' and a bit like being a 'game piece in a chess board'. She remembers some of these hallucinations quite fondly, like the time he was the leader of an all-female circus troupe and her irritation at the two faces who kept popping into her vision and asking her to wake up, because she did not want to be interrupted, she wanted to go back to the circus! Mandy would later come to recognise these faces as the medial team who were looking after her in the ICU.

One of Mandy's strongest memories from this time was when a nurse called Helen decided to undertake the massive task of taking her outside to get some fresh air and look at the sky. After six weeks in the ICU, Mandy's mental health was significantly impacted, and she was struggling to comprehend what life was going look like for her outside the hospital.

Mandy: 'I was outside, under this tree, and I saw a little bird and just had this realisation that life is so precious and I wanted to keep living it. People kept reminding me about my girls and that I had to keep fighting for them. But I think this is just who I am. I couldn't even think about the girls or my parenting duties on the other side when I was at my sickest, I just had to focus on surviving. I was surviving for myself!'

Mandy spent a total of ten months in hospital before returning home to her family, and she quickly realised they all had some big adjustments to make. She went from being the busy mum running around after her family and keeping everything in order, to having her wheelchair parked next to a kitchen bench and watching on like an observer. Rather than helping everyone else, Mandy was constantly having to ask for help. Husband Rod became her carer, and there was no denying that her relationships with her children had shifted. But Mandy was not just determined to survive, she wanted to thrive! Through a mix of dark humour and stoicism, Mandy navigated this new version of her life and nearly a decade later, she can't believe where she has ended up.

Mandy now lives in Melbourne through the week with her oldest daughter Sam who needed to relocate to complete her education. In the early days she could never have imagined living independently, but now it's just her life. Her podcast, *Look, Mum, No Hands*, tells the story of how she left the safety of her husband and carer Rod to live independently and the challenges that she faced along the way.

Mandy: 'How do you set up a house with no hands? How do you go to the bathroom in the middle of the night with no hands or feet and nobody to catch you if you fall? How do you make friends?'

Documenting this experience inspired her to extend her role as a disability advocate and Mandy's focus now is increasing the visibility of people with disabilities and opening up the narrative around people being recognised for their achievements and contributions to society, being very separate to their disabilities.

Mandy: 'Not all disabled people are going to be Paralympians! I didn't run before my disability and I'm not about to start now! Show me doctors, artists, teachers, people from all professions and experiences. Disability is about so much more than whether there is a ramp instead of stairs for a wheelchair, and people are not their disability. I do a lot of writing. And now I wonder if I even write about disability.'

Mandy knows the importance of peer support and having others to share your challenges with. When she found some other quad-amputees in Australia, she organised to meet them and their families. After this meeting, she created The QuadSquad, the first international support group for those who have had all their limbs amputated. She offers peer support to its members in Australia. She is also the founder of Get Started Disability Support Australia where she helps others living with disability. Mandy explains that when she first came home from rehab, she didn't know anyone living in a wheelchair. With three young kids, she simply wanted to take them to the movies by train, but unfortunately, she had no idea how to get there or who to ask for advice. She now created this program that covers all aspects of living with a disability.

She has travelled internationally with her family, and never one to shy away from a challenge, she has recently taken up rock-climbing. All things that would never have been possible without all the blood she received during her fight to survive sepsis and the subsequent surgeries that followed.

Mandy: 'We were in America for Halloween a few years ago and we were the best outfit in the entire neighbourhood! I had blood dripping from where my arms should have been, my husband had my prosthetic arm hanging around his neck. It was such a proud moment for us as a family … we've always used humour and stoicism to navigate challenges.'

As Mandy describes it, there is no doubt that she would be 'six feet under' without the huge amounts of blood she received. Her survival has not only given her more time with husband Rod and their three daughters but has seen Mandy achieve great success as a writer, podcast host, disability advocate, peer supporter to other quad-amputees and business owner. All of this is only possible thanks to Australian blood donors, and she offers them this message:

'Thank you! Please donate blood for me, I can't do it anymore as I have no access points! As that little bird on the branch said to me, "The life worth living is just so magical!" and if you can help someone else to do that, it's just so worthwhile, so please donate blood.'

CHAPTER 19

ELANA, JESS & JOHN

Elana Morrow and Jess Coombe are the co-founders and chief executive officers of the Accessibility, Sensory Needs and Inclusivity Index (ASI Index). They are on a mission to create the benchmark for accessible tourism and support people with disabilities to access more community settings. Their work is inspired and informed by Elana's brother John who is a blood product recipient and lives with a disability.

Elana: 'Without Australian blood donors, John would not have been able to have his treatment. Before he relapsed, he had some amazing experiences and was able to travel. We also had some really special time together in Bathurst and I got to enjoy having my big brother back. His experience inspires and informs much of our work at ASI Index.'

Jess is a blood donor and exercise physiologist with a passion for inclusivity, particularly for people with visible and invisible disabilities. Elana is a physiotherapist and has lived experience in seeing the challenges that people with disability face in accessing community settings, particularly when they are travelling and may be unfamiliar with venues they are accessing. Jess and Elana worked 'shoulder-to-shoulder' in the rehabilitation unit of the Sunshine Coast University Hospital, Queensland, and as they were supporting their patients to access the community, they dreamed about a central place where information about accessibility could be found. And when they couldn't find what they needed, they created it.

Jess: 'We've developed the Accessibility, Sensory Needs and Inclusivity Index to assist venues to communicate what they offer for people with visible and invisible disabilities. Our mission is to make accessibility information more visible and easily accessible. It's currently a website but it will become an application and all the information will be in a central location.'

When Elana talks about her brother John, it is of a childhood that so many country kids from rural Australia would recognise – growing up on a farm where they worked hard and made their own fun. Imaginations occupying their time as they went on adventures in the paddock and as they got older, on motorbikes. Country kids have a different sense of independence and responsibility for themselves but also for the land and animals around them.

This all changed when they were in high school and John was diagnosed with cancer, requiring surgery, chemotherapy and blood products.

John was in remission for two years, and during this time, he travelled to Italy, enjoying the freedom, exploration and identity-seeking activities that every young adult deserves. Experiences that would not have been possible without the blood products he received as part of his first treatment regime.

Elana: 'Before he got sick, we lived a very active lifestyle on the farm, and we were teenage siblings so we would give each other heaps! That all changed when he got sick. But when he was in remission he got back to riding motorbikes, he loved being in the country, so he moved to a place out the back of Bathurst and got a dog that he named Diesel. He travelled to Italy twice. There were some really good times and he got to really live his life. I got to hang out with him in Bathurst and that was really special.'

Sometimes loved ones of blood product recipients give examples of huge milestones or life achievements that they were able to share with their loved one who required blood and give gratitude for having them in attendance. This may be a wedding, graduation, birth of a child or funeral. Life events where the absence of a loved one may be felt most acutely. For Elana, she is most grateful to blood donors for giving her the quiet moments of sibling intimacy, where so much can go unsaid. She speaks of time outdoors together as a reminder of the carefree days outside in childhood, exploring and sitting uninterrupted on a granite rock, chatting in the sunshine and feeling that complete safety and contentment of sibling love. It's the quiet moments with her brother that Elana is the most grateful to blood donors for gifting them both.

Elana: 'When I was eighteen and just about to move to Queensland to study physiotherapy at university I decided to hop on a train and head back to Bathurst to spend three days with my dad and my brother, John. It was a difficult time, but John made me feel so safe ... I just needed to have my big brother all to myself ... I'll never forget a blissful ten minutes sitting under a giant granite boulder with my brother. I have no idea what we spoke of, I can only recall the feeling of peace and gratitude for that moment in time ... It's not as heartwarming as a wedding or birthday but it was ours and no-one else's.'

John was in remission for two years before his cancer returned and he then sustained a medical injury and developed central pontine myelinolysis, which causes demyelination of his brain. John now lives with a brain injury and disability. He has both inspired and informed so much of the development of the ASI Index.

Through their lived and professional experience, Jess and Elana conceptualised a platform where people with disability and their carers could access the community and public spaces with the confidence of knowing what facilities would be available to them at any given venue. A user may need to ensure that a venue has disability parking, a disability bathroom, no stairs, a grassy space to toilet a service dog or a sensory room. These are the types of accessibility factors that the ASI Index maps.

Jess and Elana also work with businesses to assess their accessibility and make suggestions for what they could do to make their business more accessible. They are passionate about inclusivity, sustainability and collaboration to benefit everyone in the community. They want to ensure that people living with disability celebrate their identity and culture and can access the community without the fear of barriers to access when they arrive at a venue.

Jess: 'We don't just give information to people with disabilities, we support businesses with strategies and solutions to make their businesses more accessible. Often, these are low-cost solutions and businesses want to do the right thing, they just need some guidance and support on how to make it happen and how to share that information.'

Elana and Jess both speak of choosing the professions of physiotherapy and exercise physiology and choosing to work in rehabilitation because of their deep desire to help people. But in building their business, they both really wanted to see how they could scale that so their skills, as well and their professional and personal experiences, could help a broader range of people and build the capacity of those around them to do the same.

Elana: 'We are creating something that supports people's health and wellbeing while also fostering connections, especially following COVID-19, we wanted to help vulnerable people get back out into the community.'

Everything that Jess and Elana do at ASI Index is underpinned by their philosophy of being 'being Aussies that want to help out their mates', and this is also reflected by Jess being a blood donor. Their final message to Australian blood donors is one of thanks, particularly for making Elana's brother John's treatment possible and a request for all Aussies to remember that only 4% of people living with disability are in wheelchairs. There is such a broad range of visible and invisible disabilities and the best that we can all do is choose respect and kindness.

CHAPTER 20

HOLLY & DEAN BUTCHER

To all Holly's friends:

It is with great sadness that we announce Holly's passing in the early hours of this morning. After enduring so much, it was finally time for her to say goodbye to us all. The end was short and peaceful; she looked serene when we kissed her forehead and said our farewells. As you would expect, Holly prepared a short message for you all.

Dean Butcher shared this post with the friends, family and loved ones of his little sister Holly on 4 January 2018 announcing her passing. Holly had Ewing's sarcoma, a rare form of bone cancer, and while she contemplated the end of her life, she wrote some advice that she asked Dean to post on her behalf when she passed away. Her farewell to loved ones read:

A bit of life advice from Hol:

It's a strange thing to realise and accept your mortality at twenty-six years young. It's just one of those things you ignore. The days tick by and you just expect they will keep on coming; until the unexpected happens. I always imagined myself growing old, wrinkled and grey – most likely caused by the beautiful family (lots of kiddies) I planned on building with the love of my life. I want that so bad it hurts.

That's the thing about life; it is fragile, precious and unpredictable and each day is a gift, not a given right.

I'm twenty-seven now. I don't want to go. I love my life. I am happy. I owe that to my loved ones. But the control is out of my hands.

I haven't started this 'note before I die' so that death is feared – I like the fact that we are mostly ignorant to its inevitability. Except when I want to talk about it and it is treated like a 'taboo' topic that will never happen to any of us. That's been a bit tough. I just want people to stop worrying so much about the small, meaningless stresses in life and try to remember that we all have the same fate after it all so do what you can to make your time feel worthy and great, minus the bullshit.

I have dropped lots of my thoughts below as I have had a lot of time to ponder life these last few months. Of course, it's the middle of the night when these random things pop in my head most!

Those times you are whinging about ridiculous things (something I have noticed so much these past few months), just think about someone who is really facing a problem. Be grateful for your minor issue and get over it. It's okay to acknowledge that something is annoying but try not to carry on about it and negatively affect other people's days.

Once you do that, get out there and take a freaking big breath of that fresh Aussie air deep in your lungs, look at how blue the sky is and how green the trees are; it is so beautiful. Think how lucky you are to be able to do just that – breathe.

You might have got caught in bad traffic today or had a bad sleep because your beautiful babies kept you awake or your hairdresser cut your hair too short. Your new fake nails might have got a chip, your boobs are too small or you have cellulite on your arse and your belly is wobbling.

Let all that shit go. I swear you will not be thinking of those things when it is your turn to go. It is all SO insignificant when you look at life as a whole. I'm watching my body waste away right before my eyes with nothing I can do about it and all I wish for now is that I could have just one more birthday or Christmas with my family or just one more day with my partner and dog. Just one more.

I hear people complaining about how terrible work is or about how hard it is to exercise – be grateful you are physically able to. Work and exercise may seem like such trivial things ... until your body doesn't allow you to do either of them.

I tried to live a healthy life, in fact, that was probably my major passion. Appreciate your good health and functioning body – even if it isn't your ideal size. Look after it and embrace how amazing it is. Move it and nourish it with fresh food. Don't obsess over it.

Remember there are more aspects to good health than the physical body. Work just as hard on finding your mental, emotional and spiritual happiness too. That way you might realise just how insignificant and unimportant having this stupidly portrayed perfect social media body really is. While on this topic, delete any account that pops up on your newsfeeds that gives you any sense of feeling shit about yourself. Friend or not. Be ruthless for your own wellbeing.

Be grateful for each day you don't have pain and even the days where you are unwell with man flu, a sore back or a sprained ankle, accept it is shit but be thankful it isn't life-threatening and will go away.

Whinge less, people! And help each other more.

Give, give, give. It is true that you gain more happiness doing things for others than doing them for yourself. I wish I did this more. Since I have been sick, I have met the most incredibly giving and kind people and been the receiver of the most thoughtful and loving words and support from my family, friends and strangers – more than I could I ever give in return. I will never forget this and will be forever grateful to all of these people.

It is a weird thing having money to spend at the end, when you're dying. It's not a time you go out and buy material things that you usually would, like a new dress. It makes you think how silly it is that we think it is worth spending so much money on new clothes and 'things' in our lives.

Buy your friend something kind instead of another dress, beauty product or jewellery for that next wedding. 1. No-one cares if you wear the same thing twice. 2. It feels good. Take them out for a meal, or better yet, cook them a meal. Shout their coffee. Give or buy them a plant, a massage or a candle and tell them you love them when you give it to them.

Value other people's time. Don't keep them waiting because you are shit at being on time. Get ready earlier if you are one of those people and appreciate that your friends want to share their time with you, not sit by themselves, waiting on a mate. You will gain respect too! Amen, sister.

This year, our family agreed to do no presents, and despite the tree looking rather sad and empty (I nearly cracked Christmas Eve!), it was so nice because people didn't have the pressure of shopping and the effort went into writing a nice card for each other. Plus, imagine my family trying to buy me a present knowing they would probably end up with it themselves ... strange! It might seem lame, but those cards mean more to me than any impulse purchase could. Mind you, it was also easier to do in our house because we had no little kiddies there. Anyway, moral of the story – presents are not needed for a meaningful Christmas. Moving on.

Use your money on experiences. Or at least don't miss out on experiences because you spent all your money on material shit.

Put in the effort to do that day trip to the beach you keep putting off. Dip your feet in the water and dig your toes in the sand. Wet your face with salt water.

Get amongst nature.

Try just enjoying and being in moments rather than capturing them through the screen of your phone. Life isn't meant to be lived through a screen nor is it about getting the perfect photo ... enjoy the bloody moment, people! Stop trying to capture it for everyone else.

Random rhetorical question. Are those several hours you spend doing your hair and make-up each day or to go out for one night really worth it? I've never understood this about females.

Get up early sometimes and listen to the birds while you watch the beautiful colours the sun makes as it rises.

Listen to music ... really listen. Music is therapy. Old is best.

Cuddle your dog. Far out, I will miss that.

Talk to your friends. Put down your phone. Are they doing okay?

Travel if it's your desire, don't if it's not.

Work to live, don't live to work.

Seriously, do what makes your heart feel happy.

Eat the cake. Zero guilt.

Say no to things you really don't want to do.

Don't feel pressured to do what other people might think is a fulfilling life ... you might want a mediocre life and that is so okay.

Tell your loved ones you love them every time you get the chance and love them with everything you have.

Also, remember, if something is making you miserable, you do have the power to change it – in work or love or whatever it may be. Have the guts to change. You don't know how much time you've got on this earth so don't waste it being miserable. I know that is said all the time, but it couldn't be more true.

Anyway, that's just this one young gal's life advice. Take it or leave it, I don't mind!

Oh, and one last thing, if you can, do a good deed for humanity (and me) and start regularly donating blood. It will make you feel good with the added bonus of saving lives. I feel like it is something that is so overlooked considering every donation can save three lives! That is a massive impact each person can have, and the process really is so simple.

Blood donation (more bags than I could keep up with counting) helped keep me alive for an extra year – a year I will be forever grateful that I got to spend here on Earth with my family, friends and dog. A year I had some of the greatest times of my life.

... 'Til we meet again.

Hol

Xoxo

When Dean shared this letter from Holly on Facebook, it took on a life of its own, very quickly going viral and gaining recognition and media attention in Australia and around the world. One of Holly's dying wishes was for Dean to become a blood donor and to continue her blood donation advocacy. He continues to fulfil this wish as a way of maintaining a connection to his sister and to give other families the gift of more time with their loved ones in the same way blood donors gifted him more time with Holly.

Dean describes Holly, his only sibling, as very active and sporty. He reflects on a childhood in the country town of Grafton, New South Wales, as very privileged due to the ease and freedom they experienced. He remembers them riding bikes together, visiting school friends and training a lot for sport, particularly Holly who was very talented at hockey and squash. His favourite childhood memories are of fishing, swimming, family holidays, road trips and camping at the beach, however, as with most siblings there was a healthy dose of 'squabbling', Dean remembers his mum branding him 'the shit-stirrer' and Holly 'the whinger'.

As they navigated their teenage years, Holly and Dean remained close and even both moved to Brisbane to complete their studies after school. While they didn't see each other every day, Dean says that there was never a day that they weren't in contact, be it through a phone call or a text message.

Holly started mentioning to Dean that she was tired, had some nausea and sore knees. Random symptoms that often seemed unrelated and multiple times doctors reassured her that she had nothing to worry about. In November 2016, this random compilation of symptoms was accompanied by a lump that Holly found in her abdomen, and she knew straightaway something wasn't right. Despite doctors remaining unconcerned, Holly demanded a biopsy, and the news wasn't good. Her diagnosis was rare and there was no clear treatment protocol, meaning that her treatment needed to be appropriated from another cancer type.

Dean: 'In a way, the cancer wasn't so much a shock as she had been unwell for a little while, but it was the diagnosis that she received was a stage four Ewing's sarcoma that shocked us the most. We knew that a stage four diagnosis really wasn't good.'

From this point, Holly's life completely changed. Up until her diagnosis, she was extremely fit and active, she had just completed her Bachelor of Nutrition and Dietetics and had just commenced work in the oncology department at a hospital. Holly was diagnosed on 31 October 2016 and lived for fifteen months, passing away 4 January 2018.

Dean: 'It wasn't a lot of time, if you look at the average life expectancy for a woman born now it's eighty-five years old, so she didn't even get to live a third of her life. She and her partner Luke had just purchased a house and I'd say they were gearing up to start a family in the future. But two days after diagnosis she had to start treatment due to the metastases.'

When Dean reflects on those fifteen months from that time of diagnosis to Holly's passing, he remembers her being at the hospital 'every day or two having a different concoction of drugs' and she needed hundreds of blood transfusions during her treatment.

Dean: 'From her time of diagnosis, Holly lived for about 450 more days. She would go up to the hospital and have to wait there for hours and hours, because not enough people had donated the platelets that she needed to stay alive. If you only have a fixed number of hours left on this planet, you don't really want to spend them sitting around a hospital and just praying that a stranger has had the generosity and kindness to donate the platelets that you need to preserve your life.'

At Holly's dying request, Dean is still a regular blood donor. He shares the story of his family to encourage new donors and help people to understand that the power of a blood donor is to 'save lives, improve lives and prolong lives and to feel bloody great to walk out of there knowing that you have helped someone'.

One of the most special times of Dean's life was Holly's last two weeks on this earth. He spent hours laying on a bed with Holly and chatting about their lives and her inevitable upcoming death. Asking her what she wanted her legacy to be and if there was anything that he could do to support that. Holly's response was that she just wanted to live a life of mediocrity and didn't want to cause a fuss, but she told him about a letter of farewell that she had written to her family and friends and asked her brother if he would send it when she died. Of course, he agreed, but when he asked how she wanted it to be distributed she told him that was up to him and then asked if he wanted to read it now and give her some feedback. With some minor updates and alterations over the following two weeks, that letter would be what Dean would post on Holly's Facebook after announcing her passing on 4 January 2018. They could never have imagined the response.

Dean: 'I checked the post later that night and thousands of people had both read it and shared it. I'd never gone viral before so I didn't realise how quickly it could grow. It was being reported on by the Australian media and the *USA Today*, it was even picked up by the US Secretary of State. I checked it again recently and it's been shared hundreds of thousands of times so it must have been viewed by millions of people by now. It's so ironic that she just wanted mediocrity and went viral instead!

And the key message in it was about donating blood.'

Dean says that after they finalised her letter to friends and family, Holly's next request was that he write and deliver her eulogy at her funeral. His response was, 'Of course, but you will need to give me some feedback on that too!' Dean's first draft was met with his sister's critique:

Dean: 'She said, "It's good, but it's not what you need to say on the day. You've just written about our childhood together but not enough about my life. You haven't included enough about blood donations, you need to put more in about that."'

Holly went on to explain to Dean that he needed to overcome his phobia of needles and start donating blood. He promised his sister that he would do that for her, and he has been a committed blood donor and blood donation advocate ever since. When he spoke at her funeral, he told the massive crowd: 'You probably aren't going to remember much of what I've said today because we are all just too upset, but make sure the one thing you do remember is that Holly relied on blood donations and you need to get out there and donate blood.'

Following her message going viral around the globe, Dean received messages and photos from people all over the world, particularly in the USA, who have become blood donors or organised blood donation drives after reading Holly's words. He says that from all the negativity and pain of her passing, thousands of people from all over the world have been inspired to make blood donations after connecting with her advice and her story, and that brings his family a great sense of comfort knowing that she has made such a lasting impact on the world.

Dean's message for Australian blood donors and anyone who

is considering donating for the first time: 'I have a real fear of needles and a long history from childhood of the way this phobia has affected me. But when you go into a centre to donate, they treat you like a king or queen, they are so good at what they do, and they are so professional and kind. So don't delay donating, the time is now. You can't buy happiness, but this is about as close you can get.'

CHAPTER 21

KELLIE FINLAYSON

Kellie is a mother, model, marathon runner, blood donor and blood product recipient. She and her husband Jeremy are parents beautiful two-year-old Sophia. Raising her is a juggle of commitments as Jeremy plays AFL professionally for the Port Adelaide Football Club while Kellie is undergoing a gruelling regime to fight stage four colorectal cancer. Kellie is extremely grateful to the Australian blood donors who have given her treatment options and have helped to extend her life.

Kellie: 'I am really committed to raising awareness about colorectal cancer because it's not one of the "sexy cancers". Nobody wants to talk about the cancer up your bum!'

Kellie was twenty-one, living in her hometown of Adelaide when she took her friend to see a Justin Bieber concert in Sydney and she met someone special named Jeremy. When she met him, she didn't even realise he was a professional footballer. Kellie went off and travelled the world but as soon as she got back, she reconnected with him, and they have been inseparable ever since!

Kellie moved to Sydney to be with Jeremy, and before long the COVID-19 pandemic hit, and for the AFL players and their loved ones, this meant a few years of 'player hubs' where the teams and their partners of one club would book out a whole hotel and they were not able to leave or interact with anyone outside that 'hub' unless the players were going to games or training. Kellie reports that there was no talk of getting married, but inside the hub there was lots of talk about babies in those years. Kellie and Jeremy are so lucky they planned to have a baby first and think about getting married when the pandemic was over, because they couldn't have known that Kellie had a terminal cancer diagnosis just around the corner.

Kellie's pregnancy with Sophia was far from what she'd imagined the birth of their first child may look like. They were in the hub again for the second season, quarantining with the other GWS Giants players and their loved ones in hotels as they attempted to keep that AFL season running. There was no nesting and setting up a nursery to bring a newborn to, and when precious baby Sophia was born, Jeremy didn't play for the rest of the season as he stayed in quarantine in Queensland with his newborn daughter and new mum, Kellie. They were so thrilled to be parents and so excited for their future together.

When Sophia was four weeks old, Kellie posted the following on Instagram accompanied by stunning photos of her and Jeremy with baby Sophia:

One month of you, one month of us, one month of parenthood, one month of watching my two biggest loves become best friends. It certainly hasn't been easy, the biggest life adjustment that we've ever experienced, but I do thank my lucky stars that your daddy and I get to do it all together. Best month of our lives.

However, within weeks, Kellie would be left wondering if in fact she and Jeremy would 'get to do it all together' or whether Jeremy would be raising Sophia alone as a single father and widower.

Kellie: 'My gosh, was I kidding myself if I thought that month was a hard month! That was a breeze, I had no idea that I was about to lose my first year of parenting to having treatment.'

Sophia was just twelve weeks old when Kellie was diagnosed with stage four colorectal cancer. Following Sophia's birth, Kellie had noticed an increase in fatigue, some lower back and abdominal pain and discomfort and a change in her bowel habits – all of which seem perfectly standard things for anyone who had just experienced pregnancy and birth! Especially given the COVID-19 lockdowns meant that she was not able to see a pelvic floor physiotherapist post-birth. Kellie says that while she noticed these things, it was more in hindsight that she put the pieces together. She was a new mum, and her focus was on looking after her new baby girl, not tracking her bowel and toileting habits! But it was Jeremy who finally made her make an appointment with her doctor after what started out as a bit of a joke and some banter became something he was concerned about for his wife. He was quite concerned about the frequency that Kellie was going to the toilet, feeling like she needed to poo but not being able to get anything out. They could never have imagined that the reason she was unable to go was because she had a massive tumor that was obstructing her from opening her bowels.

Kellie: 'I genuinely thought I was just postpartum! I knew for quite some time that something wasn't quite right, but also, I'd never had a baby before so I didn't really know. And I certainly didn't think that it was bowel cancer.'

Jeremy was already in trade talks to leave the GWS Giants and move to Port Adelaide before Sophia's birth and before Kellie's cancer diagnosis, so by the time she was diagnosed they were luckily living in Adelaide with the support of Kellie's family and childhood friends. This is a part of their story that the Finlaysons will be forever grateful for as it meant that Jeremy could continue his professional sports career and know that Kellie and Sophia would be well looked after by Kellie's family when he had to travel to play games interstate with the Port Adelaide Football Club.

Kellie commenced chemotherapy two weeks after her initial diagnosis, leaving no time for an egg collection as an insurance policy to the possibility of them having another baby in the future. During this two-week period, she had two major surgeries, and during the second, she lost a life-threatening amount of blood, and she was saved by Australian blood donors. Without these blood transfusions, Kellie would not have even made it to her first chemotherapy treatment. Like many cancer patients, she has also needed platelets during her treatment.

Kellie: 'Colorectal caner is just not a sexy cancer. Breast cancer – sexy cancer. Testicular cancer – sexy cancer. Even at school people will openly talk about your skin and how to protect it but nobody talks about your butt. Unless it's somebody's lovely peachy butt, but nobody talks about the actual intensive. Which I get, it's a bit of a disgusting conversation to have but it's such an important one!'

Kellie is now on a mission to raise awareness about bowel cancer and to get people talking about their bowel habits. She wants people to know what is normal and when you should be alert to changes and see your doctor. Kellie joined the Trust Your Gut campaign as an ambassador to the Jodi Lee Foundation, and in 2023 she launched an interactive symptom checker tool to recognise the signs and symptoms of bowel cancer because early detection is so vital to treatment outcomes.

Kellie: 'I have a scan next week, and I'm far from out of the woods yet. Maybe Jez will be a single dad raising Sophia alone. We just don't know. But also she's a toddler and she's a lot, and sometimes I just want some space but then I feel so guilty because I think about the fact that maybe I don't have much time left with her.'

For the Finlaysons, they are just taking it one step at a time. Australian blood donors have played such an important role in saving Kellie's life when she haemorrhaged after surgery, giving her treatment options and helping her body recover and fight cancer. Her message to blood donors is this: 'For me, and on behalf of everyone who receives blood, a big thank you and please keep doing it! When I donated blood, I didn't understand the value in it, I just did it because it was the right thing to do! But I understand now that it is genuinely so important! It saves lives! And it improves the quality of people's lives.'

While they are deeply grateful for the success in the treatment Kellie has had so far, the fact that she is living with a terminal illness is never far from their minds and she will be dependent on Australian blood donors to help her prolong this time with Jez and Sophia for as long as possible. Australian blood donors don't just keep people alive, they keep families together and give them the gift of time.

CHAPTER 22

EMMA BOOTH

Emma was always destined to be in the saddle. Her dreams of having a horse of her own came true when as a young girl she won a competition run by the TV show *The Saddle Club* of her own pony and riding lessons. This passion would take her from local pony clubs in Australia to the stables of internationally renowned dressage rider Holger Schulze in Germany and on to represent Australia. Her passion for horses would be crucial to her rehabilitation and recovery from a near-fatal motor vehicle accident in which Emma suffered spinal cord damage causing paraplegia. Emma's life was saved by Australian blood donors and her love of all things equestrian fuelled her determination first to survive and then during her gruelling rehabilitation program. Little did she know that this incredible commitment would see her representing her country as one of Australia's most prominent and successful para-athletes and inspiring so many Aussies along the way.

Emma: 'I had so many surgeries. After the airlift I went straight into the ICU, then straight to theatre to stop the bleeding in my abdomen, then from there straight back into theatre to operate on my spine. Mum and Dad signed all the consents and paperwork, but I know that I needed blood transfusions during that time that saved my life.'

Emma Booth has always felt most at home in the saddle. Even before her injury, it offered her such a sense of freedom and independence. After winning a competition with the TV show *The Saddle Club*, Emma had a pony of her own and riding lessons, and it was quickly identified that Emma had incredible talent.

In 2011, Emma was invited to Germany to ride and train horses for the internationally renowned equestrian dressage rider Holger Schulze. With limited opportunities in Australia to ride professionally, she aspired to an international career in the future. There was no doubt that she was a unique talent, and she had her sights set on the Australian equestrian team at future Olympic Games.

In 2013, Emma was returning home from a horse show in Albury, New South Wales, when a truck jackknifed and slammed into her car and the horse float it was towing, killing two of the horses inside. Emma's life was in danger as she sustained horrific injuries including bleeding on her brain and a fractured skull, a fractured sternum and ankle, severe abdominal bleeding, a shattered back, a punctured lung and a severely damaged spinal cord causing paraplegia. This near-fatal car accident would change the trajectory of her life.

Emma: 'I wasn't driving, I was the passenger and I saw it coming and thought, *This is really happening* ... the truck had jackknifed, it was on the wrong side of the road and it was a

head-on collision ... I blacked out for a while and woke up dis-
oriented to the sound of a dog barking and the car was rocking
around, it took me a while to realise that was because an injured
horse in the back of our horse float was thrashing around ... I
was stuck that way for around an hour, and when I was freed
from the car, I was flown straight to Melbourne to an intensive
care unit and that was the worst bit for my family, waiting to see
if I survived. I'm so lucky that I did.'

Emma's dream of representing Australia in the equestrian
discipline remained strong, and this was what fuelled her determination through the next four months in hospital, gruelling
physical therapy and rehabilitation. Within two weeks of the
accident, Emma was telling people that she had her sights set on
becoming a para-athlete.

Emma accepted that she would never walk again but she
never considered the possibility of never riding again. She says
this is what got her through the challenges she had with her
mental health during those long months in hospital. Emma sustained an L2 injury meaning she still had control of her upper
body and core; she knows it could have been worse, but it still
took a huge adjustment. The mental shift for Emma came in
setting goals with her rehabilitation team to get back on a horse.
Remarkably, only seven months after her accident, Emma was
back in the saddle.

Emma: 'Looking back, I think that the passion and the
love that I had for the horses and the opportunities that the
para-equestrian world gave me really saved my life. They played
the biggest role in my mental, emotional and physical recovery.
My goals gave my new life purpose and had I not gone down

that path it would have been easy to get lost ... They completely changed my life.'

Getting back on a horse gave Emma a sense of independence and purpose and she quickly set her sights on not just riding but competing. And not just locally, but at the highest levels around the world. Her passion and desire for dressage and representing her country were far from extinguished by the accident – if anything, it fuelled her fire, and in 2014, Emma made her international debut in Hartbury, United Kingdom. Not just competing but placing in the top ten in three events! Despite this being her first international event as a para-equestrian athlete, she was the highest-scoring Australian athlete of that competition and was named as a reserve rider for the 2014 International Equestrian Federation, World Equestrian Games in Normandy, France.

Emma was selected to represent Australia in dressage at the 2016 Rio Paralympics riding her horse, Mogelvangs Zidane, and finished fifth overall. She then went on to ride him again when she was selected for the 2020 Tokyo Paralympics, making Australian history as the only horse and rider combination to represent Australia at two Paralympic Games. Emma describes the incredible emotions that she felt when she walked out of the arena after her last international competition in Tokyo on Zidane, knowing that she had done far more than made history and represented her country, she had 'danced with a soulmate', such was the incredible bond that they shared.

Emma: 'The way that I've navigated life since the accident is if an opportunity presents itself – just say yes! The fear of failure often stops people from taking opportunities ... But if you are too worried that things won't go right then you miss out on incredible experiences.'

Emma retired Zidane from international competition in 2020 and planned to spend many years spoiling him in his retirement to thank him for helping her set and achieve the highest of goals. In 2022, Emma announced that Zidane has passed away unexpectedly:

I am completely saddened to announce the sudden passing of my beloved soulmate and unicorn, Mogelvangs Zidane.

On Tuesday 8 March 2022, Zidane was taken to the equine clinic for a minor surgery to remove a broken tooth. Unfortunately, he had a seizure, couldn't be resuscitated and sadly passed away.

For those who know the extent of the journey that this horse and I have been on together, and also the role he played in bringing purpose and meaning to my life again after becoming a paraplegic in 2013, you will know there are no words to describe the devastation that I am feeling right now.

People enter and exit your life in the most mysterious of ways. Zidane came into my life when I needed him the most. I know there will be other horses that I compete on at an elite level in this sport called para-dressage. But there will never be another Zidane. No bond could ever replace the one I shared with this horse.

I will be forever grateful for the joy he brought to my life and the adventures that we went on together. He will be sadly missed, but never, ever forgotten.

RIP beautiful Zidane – I'll love you forever.

Even following Zidane's passing, Emma has continued to be one of Australia's most prominent and highly respected riders. She currently holds the role as the Australian Paralympic Team

Para-Equestrian Riders Representative, liaising with other riders and providing advice on issues that impact the sport as well as its high-performance functions. Emma has continued to represent Australia in international para-dressage and most recently at the World Equestrian Games in Germany. She is an ambassador for the Victoria Racing Carnival and volunteers her time as a disability advocate and for charitable causes.

Emma: 'I just want to say thank you to the blood donors who saved my life. I donated blood for the first time recently and it was a much more emotional and cathartic experience than I had anticipated. It really made me think of the people who donated the blood for the transfusions that ultimately saved my life. Without the people that donated that blood, I wouldn't be here today. So donating blood myself and looking at the people sitting in the chairs around me doing the same, I realised the donors who saved me did something so selfless and that it had such a huge impact on so many people's lives. If you can donate, please do it! It's so rewarding and the impact that you can have is incredible.'

CHAPTER 23

THE NORTHEY FAMILY

Jenny and Peter are both blood donors as well strong advocates for blood donation. They have two children with complex medical conditions. Ava required blood products for Guillain-Barré syndrome and baby Eli suffered neuroblastoma. Their story really demonstrates how Australian blood donors don't just keep people alive, they keep families together.

Peter: 'It was a really stressful time. Our happy three-year-old first couldn't walk and then she couldn't even sit up in bed and was wetting her pants and going back into nappies despite being toilet trained, she regressed to being a baby again. We honestly thought we were going to lose our baby girl because they didn't even know what it was ... I'll never forget the nerve conduction studies, she was only two years old, and I had to hold her down while they gave her electric shocks. It was one of the hardest things I've ever had to go through.'

Nurse Jenny and police officer Peter are both blood donors. They know how lucky they are to have all their children still living. When Jenny was eighteen weeks pregnant with their fourth child (a baby boy named Eli), their three-year-old daughter became incredibly unwell with the terrifying and life-threatening illness of Guillain-Barré syndrome. This is an autoimmune disease that rapidly attacks the body causing acute illness and muscle weakness, from the patient's immune system wrongly attacking the peripheral nervous system. This is a life-threatening condition as it can cause problems with breathing, severe infections, blood clots and the risk of cardiac arrest due to autonomic neuropathy (damage to the nerves that control involuntary bodily functions like the beating of the heart).

Jenny: 'She just woke up one morning she was generally unwell, and she couldn't walk properly. This is going from a child the day before that was playing in the creek and climbing trees, running around as normal, to being unable to hold her steadiness as she walked. It was like she was drunk; her walk was so stumbly.'

After observing Ava for a few hours, Jenny became so concerned that she called an ambulance who rushed her straight to their local hospital, and a barrage of investigations began. An MRI ruled out a brain tumour; the possibility of enlarged sinuses impacting her ears and causing dizziness and loss of balance was also ruled out. With no definitive diagnosis and Ava deteriorating, she was transferred to the Sydney Children's Hospital, Randwick. Further testing in Sydney confirmed Guillain-Barré syndrome, a rare autoimmune condition.

The treatment was intravenous immunoglobulin infusion (IVIG) which treated the abnormal reaction of Ava's immune system to stop it from producing harmful antibodies that were attacking and damaging her nervous system.

Jenny: 'After one treatment of IVIG she slowly gained her mobility back and didn't require any further treatment. She walked with an abnormal gait and has had some challenges with her digestive system, but you wouldn't even know anymore, she is a crazy, energetic child now!'

Five months after walking out of the Sydney Children's Hospital with Ava, so grateful that their little girl had overcome this horrific disease and Jenny having announced that she was 'never coming back here ever again', their baby boy Eli was born. Peter reflects that they were so excited for his birth because they were still reeling from the shock of Ava's illness five months earlier, and even though she was doing so well, they were excited to have a new baby to bring excitement, new love and simple joy to their family.

Eli was born at full-term after an amazing pregnancy; Jenny says it was her best pregnancy and she had no concerns going in to deliver him via elective caesarean-section. However, after he was born, Eli did not take a breath. Babies born via caesarean-section are sometimes slower to breath as they have not had the process of contractions to help clear fluid from their lungs. But when Eli was born, there was no breath, no crying – just silence.

Jenny: 'I was on the operating table; the sheet is up in front of me, and I didn't hear him cry. I've had two other caesareans, so I'm used to the baby being born, you hear them cry, they quickly take them away and check them out and they come straight back to me. I kept asking Peter, "Why isn't he crying? Where is he? I can't hear him crying?"'

Peter was reassuring Jenny that they were just checking baby Eli out and cleaning him up a bit, but then Jenny saw the doors of theatre fling open, people running out of the room with her baby and Peter running after them. The next thing she remembers is waking up in recovery. Jenny had become so distraught and scared that they had to sedate her in theatre so that they could complete her operation. When Jenny woke up in recovery, she was informed that Eli was in the special care nursery and that Peter was with him. When she was stable, Jenny was taken to see him, and while it was confronting to see her baby needing extra support, she was never too concerned about the long-term impact of his dramatic arrival.

Jenny: 'He had the CPAP machine helping him to breathe, a little tube from his mouth down into his tummy to feed him, cannulas for fluids, and I just could basically hold his hand. The kids and my family came to see him, we could really only stroke him, but I really wasn't worried. I just kept thinking that he would be alright.'

At about 11pm that night, Jenny was recovering from her surgery and 'doped to the eyeballs with painkillers' when she got a knock on her hospital door and a paediatrician informed her that baby Eli's health had started to deteriorate and that the Neonatal Emergency Transfer Service (NETS) team had been called to fly Eli to the neonatal intensive care unit (NICU) in Randwick. Her baby boy was being sent to the same hospital that she had walked out of with daughter Ava five months earlier, vowing that she would never return.

Jenny was unable to travel with Eli that night, and despite still being in extreme pain (physically and emotionally), she was transferred via road ambulance to the Women's and Children's Hospital at Randwick the next morning. Peter had gone ahead to be with Eli as he had become so unwell so quickly. When Jenny arrived, she found Eli intubated and in an induced coma, and she realised that their baby boy may die. So, they started planning for his funeral.

Jenny: 'On day three, while I was dealing with my postnatal hormones, we had a local Catholic priest come into the hospital and baptise Eli into the Catholic faith and then we just waited for our baby boy to die. I can honestly say that it was one of the worst times of my life.'

Much to everyone's relief and surprise, Eli survived day three! But when he was extubated, he was left with a strange wheezing sound when breathing. Investigations were performed and he was diagnosed with a floppy trachea, floppy larynx and his vocal cords were paralysed. Initially this wasn't expected to cause significant issues and was possibly something that Eli could just grow out of. But as time went on, Eli was unable to be weaned off oxygen support and he was failing to thrive (gain weight). Every breath he took was taking so much energy and he was unable to leave intensive care.

When baby Eli was five weeks old, the decision was made for him to have a surgery which could have been a tracheostomy or a nasopharyngeal airway. Jenny signed the consent for both procedures and the decision would be made at the time which one was the best option for Eli. She also signed a consent for Eli to have a blood transfusion during surgery if required.

Midway through the surgery, a doctor came to the waiting room to inform Jenny and Peter that the best option was a tracheostomy. Even as a nurse, Jenny had no idea how to care for a tracheostomy, which is a surgically created hole (stoma) that provides an alternate airway for breathing. It helps air and oxygen reach the lungs by creating an opening in the trachea (windpipe) from outside the neck. The doctor went back into theatre with Eli, and while Peter and Jenny were processing what this would mean for their son and their family, the doctor returned again.

Jenny: 'He said, "We've found a mass to the right of Eli's neck. We thought he had a deviated oesophagus but now we aren't sure what it is, and we need your consent to aspirate." He reassured us that they weren't too concerned, and we gave our consent.'

Following the surgery, Eli was in an induced coma in the PICU, Jenny and Peter were by his side when a paediatric oncologist arrived to talk to them. She informed them that she did not have the pathology results from the aspiration that was done during his surgery, but that she wanted to do a core biopsy into the centre of the mass to take more cells for testing because she was '90% sure this was a neuroblastoma, lumps and bumps on babies usually present as neuroblastoma'. Neuroblastoma is a type of cancer that starts in early nerve cells called neuroblasts. Normally these cells grow into working nerve cells, but in neuroblastoma, they grow uncontrollably and become cancer cells that form a solid tumour. The paediatric oncologist was quite confident that's what the surgeons had observed in Eli's neck. The biopsy was taken, and within a few days baby Eli was given a formal diagnosis of neuroblastoma, and it was explained to Jenny and Pete that it was a rare and aggressive form of paediatric cancer. Unfortunately, Jenny was already familiar with what the outcome of this could be as she had a cousin who had died from neuroblastoma.

During this time, Pete and Jenny relied on the kindness of family and friends to help to care for their three other young children. However, once they realised that they were potentially going to be in Randwick for a long time, they were able to access accommodation through Ronald McDonald House and access the hospital school for their oldest son. They also spent a lot of time at the Starlight Room and with the incredible Starlight Captains.

Eli underwent two rounds of chemotherapy and over twenty surgical procedures, that required blood products to be on-hand as a safety net, so although he has not required blood transfusions, these procedures would not have been able to proceed without having these blood products accessible.

Eli is now three and undergoes intensive speech, occupational and physical therapy. He still has his tracheostomy so doesn't have verbal language, but he is learning Auslan. Eli has a strong oral aversion so is unable to meet his nutritional needs through food. He's graduated from a naso-gastric tube to percutaneous endoscopic gastrostomy (PEG) tube that is inserted into his stomach through a surgical incision (stoma). He lives an incredible and joy-filled life running around (much to the amazement of his physical therapy team who were unsure if he would walk).

Despite some ongoing fatigue, some digestive challenges and a mild abnormality in her gait, Ava is no longer impacted by Guillain-Barré syndrome, the life-threatening autoimmune condition that once robbed her of her mobility. One infusion of IVIG saved her life and gave her the ability to walk again. What an extraordinary gift from Australian plasma donors!

Jenny, Peter and their four kids are back to business as usual!

Work, school, children's activities and care responsibilities. It's the simple things, like getting to tuck all their children into bed at night-time, that they will never take for granted and they are so grateful to blood donors for not just saving Ava's life, but for the making Eli's treatments possible and keeping them together as a family.

CHAPTER 24

LISA COX

Lisa Cox is a disability advocate, blood product recipient and changemaker. She had a bleed on her brain at the age of twenty-four that resulted in a year in hospital fighting for her life. The only reason that she is alive today is because of Australian blood donors. She is now doing remarkable work in disability advocacy and is committed to ensuring representation and equal opportunities for people with disabilities in Australia and around the world.

Lisa: 'I have my voice again and that's an absolute privilege! I had to learn to speak again, first by pointing to letters on a board to communicate. Now that I have my voice back, I want to stand on my soapbox and advocate for people with disabilities, because I can!'

Lisa doesn't remember the day that her life changed forever, but in the lead-up she was playing elite-level sport and had just been offered her dream job. She knows that she was twenty-four years old and at Melbourne Airport when she suffered the brain haemorrhage that would leave her fighting for her life. Lisa was in an induced coma and on life support for the first few months, and her family have told her of the huge volume of blood products that were given to her in an attempt to save her life when she suffered complete organ failure. She suffered heart attacks, pneumonia, uncontrollable seizures, open-heart surgery, a hip replacement and died twice. She then needed to have one leg, all of her toes and her fingertips amputated. The permanent damage to her brain has impacted her speech and her memory and she has lost 25% of her vision. Blood products played a huge role in the surgeries that she had.

While her survival defied the odds, the hardest slog for Lisa was during the rehabilitation phase, which even now, seventeen years later, is still ongoing.

Lisa: 'The rehabilitation phase is ongoing and there are strange things that I am still learning. I have an acquired brain injury and I can forget a conversation that I had with my husband twenty minutes ago, but still remember the words to a song from twenty years ago!

In some ways the hardest thing for me was the way that society dealt with me. I had to learn how to use this new body. I was like a toddler again at the age of twenty-five – learning to feed myself, tie my shoelaces … and in some ways that was easier than the way society treated me.'

Living the first twenty-four years of her life without disability and then learning to navigate the world in a wheelchair with vision impairment and some of the cognitive deficits that have come from her brain injury has been challenging for Lisa, but the greatest surprise for her has been the social stereotyping that people with disabilities face and the way that people don't quite know what to do with her.

Lisa describes herself as a media diversity professional who is disrupting stereotypes, challenging and changing disability representation in pop culture. She provides advice to businesses and industries in comprehending and incorporating disability inclusion into their practices and content. What she wishes that everyone knew about living life with a disability is that no two people with disability have the same experiences and challenges.

Lisa: 'One in five people have a disability and they are all so different! Get to know the person before you get to know the disability! We are so much more than our diagnosis and our big fat medical file!'

Lisa knows that she would not still be alive and that none of her work would be possible had Australian blood donors not saved her life. A few years after the acute phase of her illness and just after she became engaged to be married, Lisa required open-heart surgery and another blood transfusion. Lisa remembers looking at the bag of blood and knowing that she needed to find a way to convey her immense gratitude to the anonymous blood donors who continued to save and preserve her life. Following her wedding a few years later, she penned an open letter of gratitude to blood donors; among many places it was published by the *Huffington Post* in 2016 and quickly went viral. This letter so perfectly reflects the gratitude that I hope to convey through this book and the *Milkshakes for Marleigh* podcast, and I am grateful that she has given me permission to reprint it here:

Dear Stranger,

Thank you for helping to save my life. I wouldn't be writing this if it wasn't for you.

We don't know each other but if I met you, I'd give you a hug, shake your hand, buy you a coffee or something like that. I have you to thank that I'm here today. I don't mean to sound melodramatic, that's just the truth.

That day you decided to give blood was just another day for you. You made a last-minute decision to donate and squeezed the visit in-between grocery shopping and an important deadline at work.

But to be honest, I don't care how or when you did it. The point is, you DID it. You took a few minutes from your day which helped ensure a lifetime of minutes would follow for me.

Thank you for your noble generosity. You expected and received nothing in return except for an immense glow of satisfaction. I certainly hope that is what you experienced because it's definitely what you deserve.

I am so grateful for your kindness. You have no idea how much your generosity has meant to my family and me. You'll never meet my mum, dad, brother and sister but they also want to send their immense thanks.

They lost count of the number of times they've been at my bedside and witnessed your gift restore my fragile body. Again, I don't wish to sound overly dramatic ... that's just the truth.

My husband wants to thank you too. He's a wonderful man and I wish you could meet him. We got married a few years ago.

Amongst all the wonderful memories I have of that day and of all the reasons I had to smile, I took a moment to whisper my thanks to you, wherever you were.

I wanted to send you a photo from our wedding, but I didn't have your address – so I'm writing this instead. I really hope it reaches you.

With sincere gratitude, Lisa

If you are looking for Lisa today you will find her on stage presenting a TEDx talk, as a fashion and runway model, advising media and businesses on disability inclusion or on the hunt for good coffee, because without it, none of the other things are possible! Lisa's final message to the Australian blood donors who saved her life or anyone who is considering a donation in the future is: 'If you are thinking about it, thank you for considering it, and please go ahead and do it! And if you already have, thank you for saving my life.'

CHAPTER 25

SUMMER DANIELS

Artist Summer Daniels is the founder and creative director of Little Rae Prints, where she adds a little magic to children's spaces all over the world. Summer is a blood recipient, requiring a transfusion as a teenager to help her overcome an acute infection that would impact her fertility. She has candidly chronicled her journey of infertility and pregnancy loss on her social media channels and contributed to removing the taboo around these topics, adding them to public discussion and discourse.

Summer: 'I love being surrounded by beautiful things and creating beautiful spaces. I love being out in nature and that's where I draw my inspiration for my art – I call it my big sky energy. I hope that by sharing my story I help people to feel less alone and encourage some people to donate blood.'

Summer Daniels purposefully, intentionally and unapologetically curates a beautiful life for herself, her husband and their two little girls. It's filled with beautiful clothes, a beautiful home, magical experiences and most importantly, love. A quick glace through Summer's social media accounts could have you believing that she was just an affluent influencer, showcasing her love of the finer aspects of life. But a deep dive on Summer quickly uncovers that life hasn't always looked like this for her and that her celebration of her family and the way they live their lives is a reflection of her genuine gratitude for being alive and being a mother. Both things may not be true had blood donors not provided the blood transfusion that she needed to help fight an acute infection as a teenager.

Summer: 'When you are given a healthy dose of perspective, you see life in a whole new manner! I just focus on my family, they are my priority.'

Summer knows how lucky she is to be a mother. She describes being told that she would need to undergo fertility treatment and in-vitro fertilisation (IVF) to become pregnant as completely overwhelming and heartbreaking. One of the biggest challenges she found was the lack of accessible information from other women describing their experiences. She did not personally know anyone who had been through the IVF journey and when she was told that she would require this support to conceive a baby, she assumed that meant that her chances of ever becoming pregnant were extremely low.

Summer: 'When I got the results from my surgery, I was told we would need to use IVF to have a baby, and I thought that meant that we would be extremely lucky to ever have one. I broke down, I collapsed in a carpark sobbing, and my husband told me that even if we had to sell our house, we'd do everything that we needed to to have a family. But I still went home and started to research adoption and surrogacy and very quickly realised that even those things weren't really an option until you have completely given up on your fertility journey in Australia. The outlook felt really bleak.'

Summer speaks of the grief she faced head-on when she commenced the IVF process, and she felt an overwhelming sense of 'what's the point?' not just in doing the fertility treatment that she knew only has a small chance of success, but at that time also questioned what the point of her life was. All that Summer had ever wanted was to be a mum and look after a family. These thoughts left her feeling so isolated because she had not seen her story or what she was experiencing reflected elsewhere. She bravely started to chronicle her story and share it through her social media platforms. This included the realities of fertility treatment, recurrent pregnancy loss and the joy of becoming a mother.

Summer: 'I think that it's so important to speak. It's so common and we go through so much as women, and being told that I was going to need IVF, I was so grateful to the women who shared with me that they'd had the same experience. They were the only people I wanted to talk to, and I leaned on their stories so heavily during that time so I feel like I owe it to other women now to share mine.'

The story of how Summer found herself accessing fertility treatment in the battle to become a mother starts when she was in year ten at school and preparing for her debutante ball. She was suffering severe abdominal pain for around twenty-four hours and went to the doctor who reassured her that all was fine, gave her a 'shot in the bum' and told her to present to her local emergency department if things escalated. She was reassured that she did not have the appendicitis that she originally suspected when a week later she was still unwell, mildly lethargic and in some pain, struggling to eat, but she had not had an acute escalation of her pain or illness.

Summer made it to the debutante ball, she danced with her dad and had a wonderful night, she was tired and remembers feeling 'a little dizzy' during the photos but the night was otherwise unremarkable. The next day was when things changed very dramatically.

Summer: 'The next day was when the severe abdominal pain came on, I went to the doctor and was rushed into hospital. I found out that my appendix had actually burst, and my body was doing a really good job of fighting it. The peritonitis was isolating all of my organs in the right-hand corner of my abdomen, but my right ovary had been completely destroyed. I was told that either your body fights and wins or it slowly eats every organ one by one. With that much poison coursing through my body I don't think I had much chance of coming back from it naturally.'

Summer underwent emergency surgery to have her appendix and right ovary removed, including a clean out of her abdomen. After a few days in hospital, she was released home to rest. A few days later, Summer remembers attempting to have a shower when she was hit by a wave of excruciating pain that made her projectile vomit in response. She was screaming out for help from her mother and sister and was truly terrified about what was going wrong. After a swift ambulance ride and an emergency surgery it was confirmed that Summer had developed a secondary infection.

Summer: 'I was in hospital for three weeks and required a

third surgery. I was listening to the same few songs on loop, one of them was Wendy Matthews, "The Day You Went Away"; I was so sick I thought it was going to be my funeral song. I heard doctors explaining to my parents that my blood levels just weren't recovering but my parents were reluctant for me to have a blood transfusion, my dad offered to give me his blood, but was told that it doesn't really work like that! They were just scared for me and didn't understand the level of testing required for blood to be used. But I remember the doctors saying to my parents that if I didn't have this blood transfusion, I wasn't going to recover.'

Summer was so unwell by this time that she was in an out of consciousness, and the next thing she remembers is asking her parents when she was going to have a blood transfusion, and her parents responding by pointing to the bag of blood that was going into the cannula in her arm. And from there she started to recover.

The remarkable thing about this story is that had an Australian blood donor not made a blood donation in the days before Summer needed it at fifteen years of age, then she may not have survived and gone on to have her precious baby girls Annabelle and Everly. These are the little ladies who Summer unapologetically puts first every single day because she knows how close she came to not having them. She spends her days raising her family, renovating houses, creating beautiful art for Little Rae Prints and curating insane book week costumes and dance outfits, as one of her most prominent roles now is 'dance mum'! This is an honour and privilege that Summer will never take for granted.

Her message to Australian blood donors or anyone who is

considering donating in the future is this: 'I am so grateful for anyone who donates blood. I had placenta praevia when I birthed Annabelle so I had blood on hand for her birth, I didn't need it in the end, but I couldn't have birthed her if I wasn't available.

'Please donate blood, it's so essential! I think a lot of people see blood as just being used in accidents or chronic illness and may not realise that in a situation like mine where I simply wasn't recovering from the illness, infections and surgeries, I just needed a boost to my supply to help me recover. It breaks my heart when I see it reported that supplies are running low.'

CHAPTER 26

CARLY & TRESNE

Carly and Tresne rose to fame at the height of the reality television boom as contestants on the wildly popular cooking competition *My Kitchen Rules* (MKR) in 2014. Their fame was completely dwarfed by their daughter Poppy Grace, who captivated the hearts of people all over the world as she fought childhood leukaemia. Through sharing glimpses of Poppy's journey on their social media account, the beautiful mums shared Poppy's infectious joy and charisma as she danced her way through brutal treatments. One of the most heartbreaking realities were the limitations placed on the number of treatments that Poppy could receive due to critical blood shortages.

Tresne: 'Because we were always together, and it was just the three of us, we were always in her face! I think that's made us miss her even more, it's like we've lost a body part. I know that for so long the writing was on the wall, I don't think you can ever prepare yourself for what was in store. We could never have prepared ourselves for what was coming.'

Carly and Tresne are two beautiful women from Newcastle, New South Wales, who fell in love and started a family. It took eight years of fertility treatment, with a few breaks in the middle to be contestants on MKR, travel the world, buy a house and start their businesses called The Happiness Mission and Teacher Professional Development, but their ultimate dream of coming mothers came with the birth of their daughter Poppy Grace on 2 June 2021.

Carly: 'She really was our "miracle baby!" ... I know that some people love to plan and have gender reveals, but for us it was such a nice surprise not to know that she was a girl until the very end!'

Unfortunately, Carly and Tresne wouldn't have much time at home with Poppy before finding out that their baby girl was very unwell. By the time she was six weeks old, they had noticed some abnormal bruising, which was investigated via ultrasound but wasn't deemed to be harmful. However, over the next five weeks, Poppy really wasn't sleeping well, she became very unsettled and was crying a lot. As first-time parents, Carly and Tresne didn't have anything to compare this experience to, but when their baby girl started violently projectile vomiting, they knew something wasn't right and took her to the hospital to be assessed. On arrival, a doctor was concerned about her enlarged tummy and pale skin. Tests revealed that Poppy had an enlarged spleen and an extremely high white blood cell count.

Poppy was immediately taken to John Hunter Hospital Oncology Unit where she was prepared for urgent surgery to insert a central line to receive lifesaving blood products, however, as she was so unwell, her mothers were warned that she may not survive the surgery. After the surgery, she was admitted to the paediatric intensive care unit (PICU), where she commenced a fight for her life. Overnight, Carly and Tresne became full-time carers to their baby girl with a life-threatening illness.

Tresne: 'She was eleven weeks old the day that she was diagnosed. They said that her haemoglobin was twenty-three, anything less than eighty needs a blood transfusion. But she was still fighting the doctors! They were amazed that she was even awake with levels that low, but we noticed that if we sang to her, it really calmed her down.'

Poppy was admitted to hospital in August 2021, and they would not leave the hospital again until October. Carly and Tresne speak about the nurses being a part of their family and helping them to raise Poppy, as due to the fragility of her health, being immunocompromised and the COVID-19 pandemic, community contact simply wasn't an option. Carly and Tresne still feel torn between the heartbreak that there were so many people who didn't get the chance to meet their daughter and the relief that they didn't have to share what little time they had with her with anyone else.

Poppy Grace was diagnosed with high-risk infantile acute lymphoblastic leukaemia, which has a survival rate of less than 20%. The other factors that weren't in Poppy's favour were that she was diagnosed under six months of age, with a white cell count over 150 and she had the MLL (mixed linkage leukaemia) gene. However, Carly and Tresne made an agreement with her oncologist that for Poppy to get through this gruelling treatment, then they all had to believe that she would be in that 20% that survived. Australian blood donors made her treatment possible and significantly improved her quality of life during this time.

Carly: 'We could tell when Poppy needed blood because her heart rate would go quite high which meant that she didn't have enough haemoglobin, which is basically the red cells carrying the oxygen around her system, causing her heart to work harder, and we would pick up that she was quite pale. She also sometimes needed a blood product called albumin when she was fluid over-loaded, to help draw it back into her veins. Afterwards she would feel so much better!'

The other complication was that Poppy contacted COVID-19 in hospital and tested positive for 201 days, shedding a high viral load and being highly contagious that entire time. Following her bone marrow transplant, Poppy's body just couldn't clear the virus. This meant that all her interactions with hospital staff were with full personal protective equipment.

Carly and Tresne made her life as magical as possible by starting Christmas early and running it from November all the way through to her passing in February 2023.

One of the most beautiful memories of Poppy Grace was her little glasses. Carly and Tresne speak with joy about watching her curiosity and wonder when she got her glasses and could see the world properly for the first time. Poppy loved her music therapist, child life therapists, physio exercises and visits from the limited family that were able to meet her. What she was unable to develop due to the physical limitations of her illness she made up for in her social and emotional intelligence and her ability to dance in her bed. Alongside the trauma, Carly and Tresne ensured that she had the most beautiful possible childhood inside the confines of her hospital room.

Around three weeks before Poppy's passing, Carly and Tresne were forced to confront the reality that it was likely their baby girl was going to die. Despite not showing some of the classic signs they had seen before when Poppy had deteriorated, her mums knew something wasn't quite right and requested she have a chest X-ray. They were initially told that it was all clear but a few days later, another doctor noticed an abnormality on the images. It was decided that Poppy would have a CT scan to give greater clarity and the results were that she had a fungal infection in her lungs, two big masses of aspergils.

Tresne: 'They told us that the only thing they could do to treat her was to give her white cells and that just wasn't possible because she'd had a bone marrow transplant. So, we had no treatment options. Fungal infections are extremely dangerous for people who are immunocompromised.'

A decision was made by a doctor at the hospital to cease the use of one of Poppy's medications. Carly and Tresne protested and advocated so hard for their baby girl to stay on the medication because they knew that without it the leukaemia would become refractory and would mean the end of her life. Despite Poppy being restarted on the medication later, it was too late, the leukaemia had started to double.

Tresne: 'We spoke to her palliative care team and asked what was the worst way for her to die. What's worse to take her – is it the fungal infection or the leukaemia? They explained that the fungal infection was quite close to an artery and if it hit that she would bleed out and it wouldn't be a nice way for her to go. But if it was the leukaemia, it would be more peaceful, and she would just go to sleep.'

Carly and Tresne called in every favour to organise the most beautiful christening for Poppy just two weeks before she died. They worked with Poppy's music therapist to rewrite a version of the song 'Rise Up' with lyrics that better suited Poppy's life and included a recording of her heartbeat in the song. Their immediate families and four friends were able to attend, all in masks to protect their precious and fragile baby girl. Her cousins sang for her, creating beautiful lasting memories for the whole family.

Tresne: 'We shouldn't laugh, but there was a candle as part of the ceremony and her godmother Lori tried to bring it over for her, but Poppy was on oxygen! Unfortunately, a few swear words were said, not ideal in a church! Everyone was fine but it could have been a lot worse!'

At her christening, Poppy danced and shared her comical laugh with the people that loved her the most. Her family got to see how resilient and stoic she was, in real time, rather than through photos, videos or video calls. It was a day filled with so much joy and yet so much sadness, knowing what was to come.

On 16 February 2023, Carly and Tresne posted the following update:

REST PEACEFULLY POPPY GRACE
2 JUNE 2021 – 16 FEB 2023
The morning we lost our precious baby Poppy Grace. True to form she fought tooth and nail until her final breath. Her leukaemia took over and at her last blood her blasts were at 787,000. That fighting spirit was so prominent throughout her battle and was so evident in the last four traumatic days.

Poppy showed what it is to be grateful and happy with whatever cards you are dealt. She made the most of her time on this earth, dancing, giggling and smiling right until days from the end. She was loving and funny and nurturing. She was cheeky and empathetic. She had a heart of gold and she shone so brightly, oozing joy. We felt honoured to be her mums and we didn't take a second of it for granted, not a second. She taught us so very much in her short twenty months and we have never experienced a love as all encompassing.

We are so sorry that we have to share this with you, we know how much you were cheering her on, praying for her, donating blood and bringing her fun and joy in the many gifts she received. We know there were so many children, teens and adults alike following her journey and we don't want to hurt their beautiful hearts. Please tell them that Poppy's star is shining brightly above them encouraging them to be strong when handed adversity, and to make the most of life and all its sparkling opportunities.

Please help Poppy live on through your much-needed blood donations. The Poppy Grace Lifeblood team are fourth in the Newcastle region's leaderboard – let's get her to first position. She has encouraged so many of up to rise up and help others by donating blood, please continue to give blood in her name.

We will rise up again for Poppy – we don't know what that looks like yet – we are lost and our purpose is gone. But we'll be back soon, and we will live life to the fullest in her honour. There is good to be done from the experiences we have had, there is lots to share and lots of ways that we can make the lives of oncology kids and their parents better. Until then we can rest so we can rise up for our Poppy, forever twenty months old.

As they anticipated, the response to Poppy's passing is heartbreaking to read. There is such an outpouring of love from people who never met Poppy in person but were captivated and inspired by her infectious joy and zest for life. Within days of her passing, Lifeblood centres all over Australia received blood donations in Poppy's name, and it will be impossible to ever measure the amount of lives that she saved, prolonged and improved as her followers donated blood to show their love and support for Poppy, Tresne and Carly.

Carly: 'We feel like a shadow of ourselves, but a good conversation or a meal with a friend ... these things don't lose their joy just because something traumatic has happened to you. But it does change how you show up to the rest of the world. But when it's just us, and we are alone, that's when we share our trauma.'

Carly and Tresne speak of the change of their lives and identity since Poppy's passing and this is reflected so much in Emma Madsen's work with The Carers Club. She is based on the Sunshine Coast, Queensland, and offers tailored support for carers. Emma has coined the term 'bereaved carer' to recognise the particular transition experienced by someone who is the primary caregiver for a loved one who passes away. This recognises not just the grief they experience when their loved one dies, but also the change in purpose and identity experienced by that carer who may have spent years as a carer. Giving identity to a bereaved carer also recognises the mental load associated with the 'admin' required when someone passes away – this could be anything from informing people of the death and organising a funeral, to cancelling future medical appointments, phone plans or insurance policies. It could be sorting out and distributing possessions or selling a home, or figuring out how to return to the workforce if you have been unable to engage in paid employment (or underemployed) due to care responsibilities. An example of a consideration for a bereaved carer may be that a break from the workforce meant that the bereaved carer's mortgage hadn't been contributed to at the rate they may have anticipated or there had been no contributions to their superannuation for a period of time meaning they need to reconsider retirement plans. These very few examples are by no means exhaustive and run parallel to the extraordinary grief that may also be experienced.

Tresne: 'To go from spending eighteen of the twenty months of Poppy's life isolating in hospital with her and fighting to try to save her life to now ... you do lose your identity in a sense. You just have to focus on the things that really matter.'

Since learning of Emma's work with The Carers Club, Carly and Tresne now proudly identify as 'bereaved carers', and they are focusing on charity and advocacy work during this time. They want Poppy to be remembered through the collective positive actions of others, and alongside their blood donation advocacy, they have partnered with the Children's Cancer Research Institute to run a fundraising campaign 'in memory of Poppy', they have also used their platforms to encourage people to donate blood and the response has been overwhelming.

Carly: 'We got a call from the Lifeblood donor centre and they were so overwhelmed by the increase in donations. The people in Newcastle, Maitland, Cessnock and all around her really do get behind their own. Lifeblood were amazed that we weren't connected to one of the big organisations with the number of blood donations that were going towards Poppy's Lifeblood team tally!'

When Carly and Tresne arrived at the Lifeblood centre for

Poppy's second birthday celebration, they were met with staff with poppies in their hair, balloons and they were presented with 'Poppy Grace's Corner', a seating area of the Broadmeadow donor centre that has been decorated in a garden design and a plaque with Poppy's name, remembering the incredible impact that she made on the world while she was here and all of the lives she saves even now that she has passed away, by inspiring other to donate blood.

'We celebrated Poppy's second birthday at the Lifeblood blood donation centre at Broadmeadow, which was super special, because in Newcastle and Maitland we have the most beautiful support network. When Poppy was first diagnosed, so many people contacted us and were offering help, but we didn't even know what we needed. It was actually our oncologist who suggested that we ask people to donate blood for Poppy because there was a blood shortage and that's how Poppy's Lifeblood team got started.'

Carly and Tresne have made a scrapbook that is available for donors to read in the corner with photos of Poppy and explaining the incredible impact that blood donors had on her life; they describe it as a letter of thanks to everyone who donates from the families whose loved ones received it.

Carly: 'It talks about all the times she needed blood donors to live, especially after her bone marrow transplant, when she needed platelets every second day. She needed red blood cells every week because her haemoglobin would drop, causing her heart rate to go up, she would get pale and her oxygen levels would drop ... but as soon as she got red blood cells, her heart rate would drop within the hour, and we watched it bring her back to life.'

Carly and Tresne remain committed to spreading the love,

joy and kindness that they originally set out to share with the Happiness Project, which is all just an extension of the beautiful love that they share, it's just now targeted in a different way as they focus on fundraising for children's cancer research. In August 2023, when less than six months bereaved, Carly and Tresne showed extraordinary courage and resilience when they were keynote speakers at the Children's Cancer Institute Diamond Ball which raised $1.6 million to fund children's cancer research. Teamed with their blood donation advocacy and the impact they are having on the world, there is no doubt that Poppy Grace 'got it from her mummas'!

Carly and Tresne: 'We are part of this club that no-one wants to be a part of. We are just mums who have lost a child, we are so lost, and we are just trying to find our way back. The one thing we take away from people who have navigated that path is that we need a purpose and we want to keep making a difference, for her! Just because Poppy is gone doesn't mean that our desire to make a difference stops.

'We want her legacy to live on; she inspired so many people from all over the world, if they were having a bad day, they would look at her videos and use her as a source of resilience and strength. They would look at Poppy and see her dancing and smiling, even with everything that she was going through, it would give them strength, and we don't want that momentum to stop. That's why we want to help to make a difference by increasing blood donations because we know how important these are.

'REST PEACEFULLY, POPPY GRACE x x'

CHAPTER 27

MATEOH EGGLETON

Mateoh Eggleton is an Aboriginal and Torres Strait Islander child, born into the story of his family, culture and Country. He carries with him the song lines of his ancestors and culture passed down by generations. His dreaming is part of history, while his future is his own to shape. Australian blood donors have preserved his life and given him a fighting chance to grow up with his three siblings and his fierce mumma, Shalyn.

Shalyn: 'I watched a movie called In America *and there was this big, dark god. I said if I ever had a boy that's what I'd call him! When he was born, as soon as I saw him, I knew that was the name for my boy.'*

Mateoh is just six years old and has received blood products from hundreds and hundreds of Australian blood donors. Mateoh suffers from chronic granulomatous disorder (CGD) and haemolytic anaemia.

Shalyn: 'It's a rare immune system disease where bugs have taken over his right diaphragm eating away at his liver, lung and kidney, causing many complications.'

Little Mateoh was only two when Shalyn's mumma gut told her that something wasn't right with her boy. Before this he had been a happy little boy, attending preschool and loved playing with his friends and siblings. Mateoh had been unwell for a few weeks with flu-like symptoms and Shalyn had taken him to the doctor many times as he had been so unwell and had been sent away with antibiotics for an infection.

Following a horrible week of persistent fevers and no appetite, she took Mateoh to the emergency department of her local hospital where it was quickly discovered there was something much more seriously wrong than a common childhood virus. Within two hours of presenting at hospital, Shalyn was informed that her son's blood test results were very concerning. Mateoh was in heart failure and was given an emergency blood transfusion and intravenous antibiotics. Further scans showed that he had lesions on his liver, lung and kidney.

Within days, Mateoh was transferred to Queensland Children's Hopsital in Brisbane where his care was taken over by the oncology, infectious disease, radiology and immunology teams. This was an incredibly overwhelming time for Mateoh's family as they did not have a firm diagnosis and they did not know what to expect.

Shalyn: 'His samples were sent to America for genetic testing, and Australian teams tried to confirm a diagnosis and treatment protocol. Mateoh has undergone hundreds of ultrasounds, X-rays, MRIs, biopsies and CT scans.'

Australian teams consulted with many international specialists and finally agreed on a diagnosis of CGD, which is a genetic disorder in which white blood cells are unable to kill certain types of bacteria and fungi. People with CGD and highly susceptible to frequent and sometimes life-threatening bacterial and fungal infections. CGD was initially termed 'fatal granulomatous disease of childhood' because people with the diagnosis rarely made it out of childhood before succumbing to the disease. However, with the use of prophylactic antibiotics and regular blood transfusions, there are now options for treatment.

Mateoh's first bone marrow transplant temporarily cured his CGD but left him with haemolytic anaemia, which is a disorder where red blood cells are destroyed faster than they can be produced, and this required a second bone marrow transplant.

In December 2022, Mateoh's family were given the news that a match had been found for him in the USA and he was going to be able to have a second bone marrow transplant. This was the only option available to prolong his life. However, the conditioning required for this procedure to happen would be life-threatening.

Mateoh was admitted to hospital knowing that he would not be able to leave his room for at least one hundred days. He wouldn't have contact with anyone other than Shalyn and medical staff. Once the conditioning process commences for a bone marrow transplant it cannot be abandoned or the patient will die. Terrifyingly, as they waited for his stem cells to arrive, they received a notification that it had mistakenly been left on the tarmac in the USA and there was no guarantee if, or when, it would arrive in Australia. Or if it had been impacted by the prolonged transit.

When the bone marrow did finally arrive in Australia, it was found to have been donated by a person who was now deemed ineligible to donate due to their exposure to West Nile virus. This was something that the donor was not aware of at the time of their donation for Mateoh. The bone marrow could transfer the virus to Mateoh and he wouldn't survive it. However, if he didn't have the bone marrow, he would also die as he had already commenced the conditioning process to destroy his immune system. With the impossible choice of allowing her child to die or giving him something that may result in his death, Shal was left with no choice but to proceed with the bone marrow transplant.

Shalyn: 'Heartbreakingly, the bone marrow transplant failed. In the words of Mateoh's oncologist: he is now living in unchartered territory.'

Supported by daily blood transfusions, regular platelets and IVIG, Mateoh is currently working towards ticking as many things as he can off his bucket list. Shalyn is fiercely passionate about ensuring he gets to experience as many aspects of a normal childhood as possible, no matter what the future holds. Sometimes this is hanging out with the Brisbane Broncos, it's a walk on the beach, a zoo visit or flying a kite with his siblings, attending theme parks or his first day of year one at school (even thought it was September and school started in February), being sworn in as a junior police constable or junior firefighter. Ed Sheeran even came to visit Mateoh in his hospital room! Thankfully, Mateoh doesn't fully understand why these things happen for him, just that he is an incredibly brave little boy who inspires so many people.

Shalyn: 'Unfortunately, the bone marrow transplant hasn't done the job it was supposed to in switching off the haemolytic anaemia. The haemolysis is active and isn't slowing down. Time is limited.'

In early 2023, Marleigh met Mateoh, and their interaction was something I'll never forget. Marleigh wasn't surprised by his nasogastric tube because she has had one so many times. She walked slowly with him because I told her that it was hot and his body didn't feel at its strongest today and she said, 'Mummy, that's just like me!' Shalyn and I compared stories of our children's treatment with a medication called Rituximab and how the magic of IVIG has been the thing that has preserved and prolonged Marleigh's and Mateoh's lives. As we did so, Marleigh and Mateoh compared scars and positions of their central lines and port scars (or 'special button' and 'special line' as Marleigh so affectionately refers to hers) and they giggled about how much better having their port accessed was rather than having a cannula put in. To an outsider, these conversations may have been heartbreaking. But for families like ours, they are normalising and empowering. Finding another family and having their words and story fit the shape of your wound creates an instant understanding and bond. And how lucky we are to have those moments of solidarity. The Fisher and Eggleton families will be forever grateful for the time that Australian blood donors have gifted us with our children.

Shayln: 'Thank you to all the donors. I never knew the importance of donating until my son became sick. There are so many children like my son, so please donate.'

CHAPTER 28

MISSY

After a diagnosis of paediatric cancer, acute lymphoblastic leukaemia, nine-year-old Missy had to relocate nearly 2,000km away from her tight-knit hometown community of Malanda, in Far North Queensland, to the Queensland Children's Hospital in Brisbane. She underwent 1,460 days of treatment, one excruciating bone marrow transplant, over two hundred blood transfusions, three different cancers and will be thirteen forever. Australian blood donors gave her the gift of time, treatment options and significantly improved her quality of life for four years. Her mother Anj Middlestant has dedicated her life to helping families navigating paediatric cancer and her phenomenal blood donations advocacy through the Missy's Donors Lifeblood team.

Anj: *'Missy was like my best friend, she's like my soulmate. Even though she was only here for thirteen years, I believe she was sent to me so that I could feel that profound sense of love from her.'*

Before she became unwell, Missy was the 'typical third child, baby of the family' who just couldn't wait to get into all the things that her big sisters were doing. By the age of three, her older sisters had already taught her to read the books they were bringing home from school, and as she got older, she showed a passion and real talent for her creative pursuits. In particular, she loved practising special effects and prosthetic make-up, depicting body parts falling off or wounds. She also loved spending time outdoors, finding platypus on their property and going on adventures with her best mate Flynn and enjoying her childhood alongside friends Kobi, Kelly and Chloe in a tight-knit town called Malanda, on the Atherton Tablelands of Far North Queensland.

Missy craved learning new things and she loved being at school. Anj knew that something wasn't quite right with Missy when she was nine years old, and she was so fatigued that she didn't want to go to school. Anj took her to the doctor to have the fatigue and some digestive issues investigated, thinking maybe she had a food intolerance or coeliac disease.

Anj: 'In hindsight, I think our GP knew that it was cancer as soon as she started to examine Missy and noticed a patch of petechiae on her arm where some tiny blood vessels had burst, it just looked like someone had dotted spots on her arm with a red pen. She sent us for blood tests, and at 4pm that same day, we got the dreaded phone call from our GP, who was crying. We come from a very small town and her three sons are in our three daughters' classes at the same school.'

By 1pm then next day, they were at the Queensland Children's Hospital in Brisbane, a road distance of 1,826km and an eighteen-hour drive from their community in Malanda. This is where Missy would receive a formal diagnosis of acute lymphoblastic leukaemia and go on to spend much of the next four years. Anj explains that she wasn't surprised to hear the news that Missy had cancer. She has so much cancer in her family and had lost ten direct family members to it. A fact that would become important when treatment options were considered for Missy later down the track.

Anj: 'Most kids get their port or central line surgically inserted and then they can come and go for treatment but we were at the Queensland Children's Hospital for most of that first year, we didn't leave the first time at all for four months. Missy just kept developing profound life-threatening complications, one after the other after the other … that's when the blood products really shone through. Four times I have watched them literally save her life and that doesn't count the hundreds of times that they preserved her life and made it possible for her body to withstand the toxic nature of chemotherapy treatment.

'She wanted to be a psychologist or psychiatrist because she always wanted to work people out. She just loved learning! When she was unwell all she wanted to do was get back to school.'

Anj noticed a gap in the resources provided to help families gather medical information about their child. She developed a compendium to collate this information to help reduce the mental load of primary caregivers responsible for their child's medical information. She's currently working towards expanding the delivery of this resource to all paediatric oncology families in Australian hospitals by the end of 2024 and then plans to expand the reach to other paediatric illnesses.

Anj: 'Profound illnesses like cancer rob children of their

innocence. But Missy wanted to understand what was happening with her body and be involved in the decision-making process. The compendium allowed her to collate and review her own information. The doctors would talk directly to her, and it was so empowering.'

Treatment for acute lymphoblastic leukaemia lasts for around two and a half years. After the first year of treatment, Missy and Anj were able to move back to Malanda, returning to hospital for treatment fortnightly and then eventually monthly before finally completing her treatment in December 2018.

Anj: 'Missy and I made a decision, in room twenty-four, to just do everything that we were asked to do, we just needed to get to the end date of treatment and then this would be done. We stayed really positive and tried to make the nurses' jobs easier. I really believed that she was going to be okay, there were probably only two times in that whole four years that I thought her dying was a possibility.'

Anj describes how the incredible support of the Malanda community got her family through those horrific years. From fundraising to support the family, as Anj became a full-time carer to Missy in hospital in Brisbane, while overnight her husband became a 'single dad running a small business and looking after two teenagers on his own', to meal delivery and blood donations. The Malanda community ensured that Missy's family were well-supported and they continue to do so with Missy's Donors, to honour her life.

Missy rang the bell on the paediatric oncology ward to signify that her treatment was complete. Her cancer journey was over, and she was looking forward to life returning to normal.

The family were all living back together in Malanda and looking forward to life continuing. Anj was helping her older daughters heal their trauma around Missy's cancer and the need for the family to live apart during this time and enjoying reaffirming her marriage.

This little break from the reality of cancer only lasted for six months before Anj was diagnosed with breast cancer. Six weeks after that, Missy was diagnosed with a new cancer called myelodysplastic syndrome (MDS) which required an urgent bone marrow transplant as it can very rapidly progress to other types of cancer. Missy's sisters were urgently tested to see if they were suitable donors while Anj was scheduling in her double mastectomy to deal with her breast cancer within the time line of Missy's conditioning for a bone marrow transplant. Again, they would have to relocate nearly 2,000km south to Brisbane, but luckily Anj could have her surgery at the Mater, across the road from the Queensland Children's Hospital.

Anj doesn't like to identify as a 'cancer survivor'. All three of her cancers have been found early, surgically removed and no further treatment has been required. In all, it was found that she had breast, uterine and bowel cancer. Due to the sheer volume of cancer within Anj's family, genetic testing was undertaken that revealed Li-Fraumeni syndrome. Which is a rare, autosomal dominant, hereditary syndrome that predisposes carriers to cancer development. It comes with the complication that radiation cannot be used as treatment as it increases the risk of secondary and tertiary cancer development.

Anj: 'For some reason my thirteen-year-old daughter experiences four years of pain and heartache and dies, and yet I have three different cancers and they are all just cut out, no further treatment required. I didn't have chemotherapy and I couldn't have had radiation because of a genetic diagnosis in my family.'

Test results revealed that Missy and her older sister, Freya, were both Li-Fraumeni syndrome carriers while their big sister Amelia was not. This was incredibly lucky as it was Amelia that was a match and the donor for Missy's bone marrow transplant, which while fraught with complications, gave Missy a chance to fight MDS. One of the biggest complications Missy faced was when she started bleeding internally in her lungs, she was unable to have the coagulation medication as it would harden the blood in her lungs and kill her. She was moved to the paediatric intensive care unit and not expected to survive. A creative solution was developed by a doctor to turn the coagulation medication into a gas and administer it to Missy through a nebuliser. Within three days, the lung complication had been reversed but Missy's platelet numbers were incredibly concerning.

Anj: 'During that time, Missy's platelet numbers were in the single digits. A healthy person has a count around two hundred. Missy's were being tested twice daily and coming in at two, then five, then zero. We had a two-and-a-half-week period where Missy was receiving one bag of platelets every six hours. To make one bag of platelets, it requires four people to make a whole blood donation and she needed these every six hours. Sixteen people needed to donate blood every day for two and a half weeks just so one little girl could keep fighting to stay alive. That's the power of blood donation.'

During her four-year battle with cancer, Missy was a vocal advocate for blood donation and for other factors impacting families navigating paediatric cancers. She was an incredible public speaker, so well-versed in her own condition and journey, she was the face of Daffodil Day for the Cancer Council and worked with Woolworths on a campaign where people could buy tokens to benefit childhood cancer sufferers. She loved going to Lifeblood donor centres and thanking blood donors, and Anj continues this tradition in her honour.

Missy and Anj kept their promise to each other and they did everything the doctors and nurses asked them to do, but when Missy was diagnosed with a third form of cancer, while undergoing treatment for MDS, Anj had a big decision to make. As they had exhausted all possible treatment options, would she tell her precious girl that after all she had been through, she was going to die? In the end, she chose to spend those final days filled with love and hope. Adding additional fear and frustration for Missy would not have changed the outcome.

Anj: 'I find death interesting in a way, I cared for my dad through his cancer battle, I was his primary carer during grade eleven and twelve, he passed away at the age of forty-two, three months after I finished high school. There is something really empowering about being with someone that you love when they pass away. It's a real gift, I can't imagine having to die alone and I don't believe that death is the end.'

Anj says that in her last few months, Missy was frail but comfortable. She was still mobile, still doing some schooling and blissfully unaware of how close the end was. But Anj could see the signs. Missy's eyes became droopy, her hair became crispy, and they were home in Malanda when she became quite unwell. They were at the Cairns Base Hopsital, in an isolation room with no windows, the staff were unfamiliar, and Anj just knew that that Missy couldn't die there. It was only the second time that Anj truly allowed herself to believe that her baby girl was going to die.

Missy and Anj were transferred back to the Queensland Children's Hospital and admitted to room four, which was Missy's favourite room and where she had received the life-preserving bone marrow from her sister Amelia. Anj was given the option of choosing the nurses that would look after Missy at the end and then had to ask all the staff, who all loved Missy so much after looking after her for four long years, to stop being so extra nice to her as she was going to work out what was going on! In the end, things progressed very quickly. Missy went to sleep peacefully and didn't wake up again. Her dad, Rob, and sisters, Freya and Amelia, came to Brisbane, but she was already unresponsive by the time they arrived.

Anj: 'We were just in her room and when she woke up that morning, she was very incoherent. I got the nurses to help me move her into the armchair so she could feel the warmth of the sun on her body, she could no longer open her eyes but I'm sure she enjoyed that warmth. Then we popped her back in her bed and thirty-six hours later, she passed away at 7:48am with Rob and me holding her hands, she took those last three big breaths … and she was in a room surrounded by so much love. The nurses that were looking after her were the same two nurses that looked after her when she was nine and was first diagnosed … She couldn't have made it more perfect if she tried, it was actually really beautiful, holding the hands of her mummy and her daddy, surrounded by love. And didn't even know that she was dying. Her last thought would have been of her tomorrow, and that's one of the greatest gifts we could ever have given her as parents is for her to believe that there is a tomorrow.'

The incredible gift that Anj keeps giving Aussies every day in honouring Missy and her legacy through Missy's Donors is the gift of a tomorrow for those who rely on blood products to save, prolong or improve their lives. Anj described her work as giving her purpose and that 'purpose in the alarm clock that gets me out of bed some days'.

Missy's life continues to be remembered and celebrated by her friends in so many creative ways. This includes her mate Kobi organising a group to push a wheelbarrow 140km from Mareeba to Chillagoe on the 'twentieth anniversary of the Great Wheelbarrow Race' in Missy's Donors budgie smugglers, which have now gone on to be a great fundraising item!

Missy's best friend Flynn, who races cars in khanacross events, has decked out his car in red paint with huge Missy's Donors stickers, and every time there is a local school sports carnival, it's impossible to miss the sea of Missy's Donors red T-shirts. So many acts of kindness, big and small, that keep Missy's memory alive, and this sustains Anj, Rob, Amelia and Freya, because their greatest fear is that Missy will be forgotten and people will stop saying her name.

Anj's final message to Australian blood donors or anyone who is considering a blood donation in the future: 'I just want them to know how important every single blood donation is. We couldn't have undergone Missy's treatment without them, but most importantly without the love and compassion in her community that carried Missy through it all.'

Finally, Anj says that some of the biggest supporters of Missy's

Donors and some of the most amazing blood donation advocates that she knows are people who can't donate blood. Anj is one of these people! And whether it's telling people about Missy, reminding people in your household to make their blood donation appointment, sharing one of Missy's Donors social media posts (listening to the *Milkshakes for Marleigh* podcast or buying a copy of this book!) it's all blood donation advocacy in action. The hope being that the complacency of the twenty-nine out of thirty eligible Australian donors who don't donate will be shifted.

Anj: 'I just want people to get in there and save some lives! The most amazing thing about blood donation is that you can't synthesise blood, you can't make blood! It must come from one human to another.'

CHAPTER 29

MICHELLE & JARRAD WEEKS

When Shane Carty became unwell, he was initially misdiagnosed before it was revealed that he was suffering from multiple myeloma, which is a rare and often overlooked form of blood cancer. Before his passing, he received many blood products that gave him treatment options, prolonged and improved his quality of life. Giving him more time to make precious memories with those who adore him. His daughter Michelle and her husband Jarrad are committed to raising awareness about multiple myeloma.

Michelle: 'My dad was a beautiful human! A giant, gentle, wonderful man! We grew up in South Africa, he'd had a very successful rugby career, but he and my mum gave up a lot for my sister and me to come to Australia and start a life that was very different but it was the best thing for our safety.

'He just had this incredible knack about him that every person he spoke to felt seen, heard and understood. Very calm, very gentle,

he had a very wide network of people who just loved him! We were lucky to have him as our dad! He was a very special human!'

Michelle Weeks is a life and mindset coach who dedicates her professional life to helping mums lighten their mental load. She has an amazing podcast called *A Mother's Mind,* where she unpacks navigating motherhood. She is mumma to Freddie Shane and expecting the arrival of their baby girl in late 2023. You can often find Michelle, coffee in hand, playing with Freddie on the sand of Blackman's Bay in Tasmania, where she and husband Jarrad are carving out a life and raising their family. Michelle is deriving great joy from having a pantry in her kitchen that she can properly set up and know that she won't be emptying it again by the end of the basketball season. She is married to recently retired National Basketball League (NBL) star Jarrad Weeks, who had an outstanding career playing in Australia and New Zealand, finishing his professional career as a foundation player for newly established Tasmanian Jack Jumpers NBL Club, with whom he accepted a coaching position at the end of his playing career. The Weeks family loved their time travelling around playing basketball but are so very excited to reduce their travel and focus on raising their young family. Family has always been the most important thing to both of them and why they are both such proud blood donors and blood donation advocates.

Michelle: 'The thing with multiple myeloma is that it's a rare form of cancer and it can for a long time be undiagnosed. In my dad's case he was misdiagnosed at the start. It a rare blood cancer that just not often on the radar.'

The signs and symptoms of multiple myeloma can include bone fatigue, pain or fractures, breathlessness, frequent infections, thirst and/or nausea. When Shane became unwell, it caught the whole family by surprise. He was a very fit and healthy man and the only signs that presented were a bit of aching around his ribs and pelvis, which felt a bit like a cramp. But when Shane had a routine scan done for his heart, some abnormal shadowing was noted. This was investigated and initially explained as being caused by 'old rugby injuries', but luckily for Shane, further investigations were done that indicated multiple myeloma. Shane had a bone marrow aspiration to confirm the diagnosis, which was initially negative, and the family were informed that no evidence of myeloma had been detected, however, further results then revealed non-secreting multiple myeloma which is so rare and does not even have a clear treatment protocol.

Michelle: 'We started the roller-coaster from there. It was seventeen months from the day that he was diagnosed to the day that he passed. His team at the Royal Prince Alfred were just phenomenal, not just for my dad and the aggressiveness of his cancer, but for my mum and my sister and me as well. I don't think any of us believed that he actually would die, we just thought it was a long-term disease.'

Michelle speaks of the incredible periods that they had in-between treatments where Shane was out of hospital and able to enjoy life. He underwent a stem cell transplant that had some benefits, but the decision was made for him to also undergo a medical trial of CAR-T cells.

Michelle: 'When you lose someone it's so comforting to know that everything possible was done to try to save them. Every single thing was done. It doesn't make the grief easier, but it does make you grateful for medicine, the system and the people that are working their butts off every day to nurse people back to health or to a place that they are as comfortable and able to spend as much time as possible with their families.'

One of the big challenges that Michelle and Jarrad faced during this time was knowing when the right time was to go to Sydney to be with Shane. This was especially tricky during the conditioning phase of his stem cell transplant as he was so immunocompromised and community contact needs to be limited. Shane lived in Sydney and at the time he was diagnosed, Michelle and Jarrad were living in New Zealand. What they couldn't have predicted was that a global pandemic called COVID-19 was about to hit the world and make all their decisions and travel that much trickier to navigate.

Jarrad: 'It was tough while Shane was going through his illness and his treatment and not getting to see him. I was playing for the New Zealand Breakers, so we played the offseason in New Zealand, and then due to COVID-19 we got relocated to Melbourne, then we got the call that it was best for Michelle to go back to Sydney so that's what she did and I went on the road with the team.'

It was difficult for Jarrad to follow COVID-19 protocols and team rules while watching the border closures and restrictions that kept changing while knowing that Michelle was with her terminally ill father. Especially as only a few days before she had flown to Sydney, they found out that Michelle was pregnant with their first child.

Jarrad: 'With COVID-19 we just got shafted every which way and I just didn't know when I was going to be able to get home. Luckily, the general manager at the club allowed me to go home for four days so that I could see him. Shane got to see my gorilla feet one more time and I'll never forget him saying that!'

Jokes of gorilla feet aside, Jarrad got to spend four days with Shane and support his wife for this time before he had to rejoin his team and 'go back on the road'. This was especially tricky as not only was he likely saying goodbye to his father-in-law, he was also leaving his pregnant wife without certainty of when he would see her again. When Shane passed away, Jarrad was unable to be physically present to support Michelle, and he had to watch Shane's wake via video link. Those four days were the only time that he saw Michelle in four months. Missing most of the pregnancy, dealing with his grief over Shane's passing while trying to support Michelle remotely and dealing with the internal turmoil of not being able to prioritise his family. COVID-19 making what was already incredibly painful, so much more difficult.

Jarrad: 'It was such a tough situation. I was stuck in a hotel room in Hobart and only allowed to leave the room for a few hours a day to practise or play basketball. I get off the phone to my pregnant wife and her dad had just died, but I have to go to practice that afternoon and try to give a shit. It was really tough on all of us. I just tried to use my time on the court as an outlet … I tried to remember that Shane wanted me to keep playing. He didn't want me to get on a plane and leave the team and Michelle kept telling me that him getting to watch me play was bringing him joy.'

Realistically, Jarrad was doing the best thing for his family during that season and into the future. Any family who has had a loved one experience injury, illness or disability knows that just because you are facing the most heartbreaking time of your life doesn't mean that bills don't need to be paid, and as a professional athlete, Jarrad needed to position himself not just for that season but for future seasons as well. Especially as he was about to become a dad for the first time.

Michelle: 'Dad did NOT want Jarrad to stop playing! Doesn't mean that it was any easier! But he loved to watch him play, even when he was so unwell he'd sit up with his T-shirt and his beer in his undies and watch a game. It brought so much joy to both our families.'

Michelle reflects on one of the most special times of the four months that she spent in hospital with her mum and sister caring for her dad was when she told him that she was pregnant with Freddie. Her sister took a video and it's now lovingly in Freddie's room as a connection between Shane and his grandson. She speaks so lovingly of this time and the photos they had around the hospital room, including ultrasound pictures of Freddie and talking to her dad about how she and Jarrad were going to be parents. These moments are gifted to families by Australian blood donors. They gifted Shane the knowledge that during his final months, his grandson was in his hospital room, nestled and growing safely in Michelle's belly. So even though he passed away before Freddie was born, Michelle got to share that experience with her father.

One of the great legacies that Shane has left in this world is the wisdom that he shared with his daughters and the loving community that surrounded them. Michelle now maintains her connection to her dad by sharing 'Lessons from Shane' through her social media. Some of those lessons are shared here with her permission:

Lessons from Shane

You actually only have the here and the now, waiting is a wasted state.

There are precious moments to snap up while others or our past selves are waiting. Embrace the now and create the best flipping life you can. It's always going to be worth it.

We don't have control over our lifespan, but we do have control every day to engage with the world in a way that lights us up and makes each day grand, despite the challenges and hurdles that are thrown at us.

Throw kindness around like confetti! Make people feel seen, heard, loved and understood.

Love life and live unapologetically as yourself!

Mic, my lovie, untie your shoelaces. You need to take care of the little things. They matter.

Drink the good wine.

Michelle: 'Dad was getting a huge amount of blood towards the end and that kept him more lucid, and for us that was such a gift because we got more time with him and people could come to say goodbye to him and he was aware of who was there.

'Please make it a part of your regular routine. Blood donors will never understand the impact that that they have. The impact on the patients themselves and time that they gift for their loved ones to spend with them. We are so grateful and appreciate the time our donors took out of their lives to gift us more time with my dad.'

Jarrad and Michelle use the lessons that Shane taught them through the way they curate their lives with such purpose and intention. They talk to Freddie about his Grandpa Shane, and how he always made everyone in the room feel seen and heard, and they encourage little Freddie to aspire to approach the world with the same grace and kindness as his moniker.

They will tell stories to their baby girl about her 'gentle giant' of a grandpa, and as their children grow older, they will encourage them to join them as blood donors. As there is no greater kindness than giving families the gift of time and there was no kinder human than Shane Carty.

CHAPTER 30

JULES

Julian is a medically discharged soldier of the Australian Army who suffers from acute disseminated encephalomyelitis (ADEM) which is a type of autoimmune encephalitis and myelin oligo-dendrocyte glycoprotein (MOG). Intravenous immunoglobulin infusion (IVIG), made from donated human plasma, is used to treat both of these conditions.

Jules: 'I've had seizures, been blind and paralysed. So, to jump in the spa and crack a beer with my girlfriend on a spring afternoon, I finally felt normal. Being seizure free for one year means I can have a bath again, I can think about driving again! I'm so grateful to Australian plasma donors.'

In December 2018, Jules was preparing to deploy to Iraq as a soldier in the Australian Army. Part of his pre-deployment medical checks included vaccinations including pertussis, typhoid, diphtheria and tetanus. He then travelled from Canberra to Sydney for a pre-deployment course where he started to 'feel funny' and experience some concerning symptoms. First, it was sinus pain, but without a runny nose. Then he noticed that he was unable to empty his bladder completely. This resulted in hospital admission and a catheter was used to drain his bladder due to concern about damage to his kidneys. Jules was discharged and travelled back to Canberra to finish preparing for his deployment.

Jules: 'The next thing that happened was that I couldn't walk properly. It was just like I was drunk. Then as I was packing my bag to leave for Iraq, I fell over, like I was really drunk and I couldn't get back up. I got myself to my physiotherapist, David Bloom, who thought I had a septic infection and took me straight to hospital.'

The next two weeks were filled with blood tests, scans, a lumbar puncture and a diagnosis by exclusion of other possibilities. During this time, Julian described himself as being in a 'comatose-like state where I was either sleeping or vomiting', he lost over 15kg during this time. His first treatment was a high dose of intravenous steroids, which made him manic and there was a clear change in his personality.

Julian: 'Then I needed to learn to walk again. There was so much nerve damage that the signals between my brain and my legs no longer worked, and I was unable to walk. I was largely unphased because the steroids made me so hungry all I wanted to do was eat! I was still quite manic and all I wanted was for someone to get me a wheelchair so that I could get to the hospital cafe to get a myself a coffee!'

Once Julian's diagnosis of ADEM was confirmed, he was able to commence treatment with IVIG and this is when Australian blood donors saved his life. As soon as he knew that he was going to live, he was ready to set and achieve rehabilitation goals. One of the great benefits to being in the military in this situation is that 'when someone tells you to do that for an hour, you do it!' and Jules made very effective progress in his hospital rehabilitation program. Once he got to his walking frame, he was off to the hospital cafe as much as he could. Then he progressed to a walking stick, and six weeks later, he was home.

Julian: 'It wasn't so much losing my ability to walk that was the problem, it was the seizures. The postictal confusion was horrible and so scary for everyone around me.'

Jules credits his survival to the incredible medical staff that supported him and his neurologist, who he trusts implicitly. And of course, the thousands of blood donors who made treatment possible for him in the initial acute phase of his illness but then to manage his severely compromised immune system in the years that followed. He maintains he couldn't have done it without the support of his mum, and the thing that motivated him the most was his best mate, Angus. Angus was a brown-and-white beagle who carried Jules through the roughest of times. He passed away unexpectedly in August 2023 and Jules shared his grief so profoundly:

Angus
Nothing is forever, for sure is what they'll say
You were always going to outlive him anyway
And I guess I always knew that was the way it would be
Me farewelling him, not him farewelling me
Years ago, I gave you a home and a name
Once I had you in my life, it was never quite the same
But yesterday I knew it was sadly the time
To take away your pain and to make it mine

I will cry, I will cry, in my grief I will wallow
If I knew where you had gone you can be sure I would follow
To give you one last pat, and have just one more day
But you have gone where I cannot, and here I'll have to stay
Without you in my life, nothing is what it seems
Until we meet again, my boy, I'll see you in my dreams.

By Julian Hohnen

The conditions of his medical discharge from the army meant that he didn't have a financial need to return to work and this was further enhanced when in 2019 he won the Lotto! This allowed him to buy a beautiful home to enjoy with new partner Alexandra, and on Valentine's Day 2023, they became engaged.

Julian: 'During my career I did six months in Timor, nine months in Afghanistan and twelve months on a UN job in Syria, so one of the things that my medical discharge has meant is that I can finally put down some roots, knowing that I'm not going to have to move every two years with the army.'

Jules didn't want to accept that at the age of forty-two he was never going to work again and rather than 'rushing to failure', he took time finding a pursuit that could accommodate the challenges he still faces. Initially, this was that he was not able to drive due to the seizure risk and 'public transport just isn't an option because I have the bladder of a four-year-old'.

Four years after the acute onset of his illness, Jules is now seizure free and back behind the wheel of a car. He is an incredible writer and has pieces published by various outlets and he appeared on the SBS program *Insight* to offer expertise on the fall of Kabul one year on and what it might mean for the veterans who served there.

Everything that happened for him – the survival, winning the Lotto, the dream house, spending more time with his loved ones like his mum and Angus, his volunteer work and blood donation advocacy, becoming engaged to Alexandra (who is a plasma donor) and returning to the workforce to build a new career. None of this would have been possible without the Australian blood donors who saved and preserved his life.

His message to them is this: 'A genuine thank you. It's a simple gesture. I've been shot at, and I hate needles and I hate cannulas but you can handle it. You get a free milkshake! For such a small gesture, it has such a marked effect on a lot of people.

'Having a lot of donors makes a huge difference. This helps people with a variety of conditions, and for people like Marleigh and me, it saves lives. I hope that telling my story and Milkshakes for Marleigh sharing so many stories, people can see where their blood goes and we can get Australian donor numbers up.'

CHAPTER 31

AMY PURLING

Amy Purling, better known at the Miracle Mumma, is one of Australia's most prominent advocates for premature babies and their families. She is the creator and host of *RAWR The Podcast* where she and co-host Grecian interview their guests about premature babies and life in the neonatal intensive care unit (NICU), special needs, infant loss and everything in-between. After facing pregnancy loss and fertility challenges, she and husband Scott are proud parents to James and Jack, two beautiful little boys who are only alive thanks to Australian blood donors.

Although she had experienced pregnancy loss and fertility challenges, Amy had no idea that her firstborn James would arrive prematurely. However, he entered the world ten weeks early at thirty weeks gestation, and overnight Amy because a 'NICU mum' to an incredibly unwell baby boy who had a rare blood disorder called neonatal allo-immune thrombocytopaenia (NAIT).

Amy: 'Basically, James inherited platelet antigens from my

husband which were recognised by my body as foreign, and I made reactive antibodies which crossed the placenta and subsequently "attacked" James' platelets in-utero.'

Despite being an emergency department nurse, this news was very overwhelming for Amy, and she remembers the neonatologist sitting with her in the NICU and drawing simple diagrams to make the complex diagnosis as simple for her to understand as possible. What she really didn't understand at the time was the scramble happening behind the scenes to source James the platelets he needed, made more logistically complicated as they have such a short shelf life. Specific donors were being called in other states and being requested to make blood donations which were then being put on ice and flown to Adelaide for James.

Platelets are a component of the blood essential for clotting. Low platelet levels cause bleeding into tissues and subsequent bruising, with severe cases causing irreversible intracranial haemorrhage (bleeding on the brain), resulting in long-term disability or death. This condition isn't routinely screened for in pregnancy.

Amy: 'James was born extremely bruised and swollen with a petechial rash caused by broken capillary blood vessels. He was found to have a severely low platelet level which was life-threatening. He immediately received a transfusion, but his levels didn't rise as expected. This is when the doctors started testing for NAIT and discovered that James required specific platelets.'

The specific platelets that James required were donated in Melbourne and flown to Adelaide. On arrival, the volume was divided very carefully into three doses that were infused over twenty-four hours. For James, this treatment was enough to kickstart his own body into producing the platelets that he needed, and he has not suffered significant long-term damage, despite having a bleed on his brain while in the NICU.

When planning their next pregnancy, the Purlings had a lot more information on their side and were able to manage Amy's high-risk pregnancy quite differently to ensure the best chance of survival for her baby if he too was diagnosed with NAIT.

Amy: 'Every week from nineteen weeks pregnant until delivery, I received five precious bottles of IVIG, a product made from human plasma and obtained from approximately one thousand voluntary blood donors. The doctor explained that these antibodies flood my blood and "trick" my body to stop creating the specific antibodies which attack the baby's platelets.'

They knew that even with Amy undergoing this treatment, there was small chance that when baby Jack was born, he would still require platelets, and unfortunately he did, but this time the NAIT wasn't a surprise and they were much better prepared. Without Australian platelet donors, neither of Amy and Scott's boys would have survived long past birth.

A message from Amy to Australian blood donors: 'I want to say a personal thank you to all those who donate blood, from the very bottom of my heart. None of this would have been possible if it weren't for the generous and selfless donors who took their time to save a life – and not just any life, but our sons' lives. Our difficult journey has been made so much brighter by the goodness of people we have never met, and we will forever be in their debt. You do not have to be rich to be generous.'

James and Jack are now joyful little boys who are relishing living on the farm that the family recently purchased outside

Adelaide. They can be found in the chook pen, riding bikes in the paddock or getting into mischief with their new Labrador puppy, Bowser.

Jack balances a number of health challenges and has a PEG for feeding. He also has monthly subcutaneous immunoglobulin infusions, which Amy administers at home to reduce his medical trauma. The family are deeply entrenched in their local community, and they can be found most weekends at the AFL grounds where both Amy and Scott play for their local team and the boys won't be far behind them.

The Purlings know that Australian blood donors don't just save lives, they keep families together.

CHAPTER 32

SNAPSHOTS

There is no way that all of the stories shared through the Milkshakes *for Marleigh podcast and community could be told within the pages of this book. Instead, I have included snapshots of these stories and the messages of thanks from blood recipients and their families.*

Chloe Wigg – Artist, disability advocate and 'undisputed queen of the nutbush'
Season one, *Milkshakes for Marleigh* **podcast**
Receives intravenous immunoglobulin infusions (IVIG) to treat multiple autoimmune conditions including myasthenia gravis.

Thanks blood donors for gifting her the 'difference between life and living'. IVIG significantly improves Chloe's quality of life, allowing her to intermittently create art, engage as a disability advocate and have the energy to sit up at the table to share dinner with her son and husband at night-time.

Adam 'BarRat' Barrat – Mental health advocate and Sunshine Coast media personality
Season one, *Milkshakes for Marleigh* podcast
Received a blood transfusion when a fall from a ladder while completing routine home maintenance left him with a broken back.

Thanks blood donors for gifting him his life so that he can see his kids grow up.

Geoff Callaghan – Commonwealth public servant
Season one, *Milkshakes for Marleigh* podcast
Geoff's little brother died of leukaemia in early adulthood, leaving behind a young son. When Geoff was diagnosed with myeloma he wondered how long it would be until his daughters would also be growing up without their dad.

He thanks Australian blood donors for making his treatment possible and giving him more time with his wife Lauren and their two young daughters. Spending Christmas morning with them after his diagnosis was magical.

Claire Devine – Artist and mother at the helm of a family with additional needs
Season one, *Milkshakes for Marleigh* podcast
Claire suffered the life-threatening complication of ovarian hyperstimulation while undergoing fertility treatment. The treatment was albumin, a blood-derived plasma product which not only saved her life but gifted her the chance to go on to have a family.

Between her husband and her sons, they have a range of conditions that may require blood products in the future, including cancer, epilepsy and albinism. Claire is grateful to the blood donors who helped her to create her family and now provide the safety net she needs to keep them well.

Brendan Hall, OAM – Swimmer, Paralympic gold medalist, surf lifesaver and 'competitive mongrel'
Season one, *Milkshakes for Marleigh* podcast
At the age of six, Brendan lost 70% of his hearing and his leg due to complications of chicken pox. He is lucky to have survived and then become a Paralympic gold medalist, however, he is most proud of his contributions to his local community, particularly as a volunteer surf lifesaver. He was awarded an Order of Australia for his contributions to Australian sport.

Most importantly, Brendan is grateful to his blood donors for gifting him the opportunity to experience becoming a husband and a father.

Tallulah Moon – Inspires everyone around her to find genetic cures for kids
Season one, *Milkshakes for Marleigh* podcast
Tallulah Moon is a fiercely independent five-year-old who can manoeuvre a wheelchair in a manner that would put most Paralympians to shame! *Our Moon's Mission* seeks to find a cure for SPG56, the neurodevelopmental condition that is impacting Tallulah's ability to walk and talk.

Tallulah's mum, Golden, is a proud blood donor, and plasma infusion remains a possibility for Tallulah in the future. Her family wants to find a cure for SPG56 and all genetic conditions impacting children. They also encourage people to donate blood so there is enough in Australia's supply if Tallulah (or anyone else that they love!) ever needs it.

Michael Jibrail – Father to a child battling cancer and blood donor
Season one, *Milkshakes for Marleigh* podcast

Michael is a blood donor and the father to a little boy who is battling childhood cancer. Through social media platform Tiny Gratitudes, he shares the realities of what children endure on their cancer journeys and the crucial role that blood donors play in making treatment possible.

Alana and TJ – Mother and son whose lives will never be the same following a road crash
Season one, *Milkshakes for Marleigh* podcast

TJ was a promising young footballer who had just completed his first year of high school when he was involved in a road crash. He was a passenger in a car his mum Alana was driving, when they were hit by a drug-affected driver.

His seatbelt saved his life but caused him to suffer a perforated bowel requiring a double stoma, the loss of major abdominal muscle, fractured ribs and a punctured lung. The only reason he is alive at all is thanks to Australian blood donors.

His life will never be the same, but TJ recently finished high school and is back playing football every weekend. Teamed with his mum Alana, they have contributed to advocacy and awareness campaigns for road safety, road trauma victims, risk-taking behaviours, the Canberra Hospital Foundation and blood donation advocacy.

Adam Cheyne – Town planner, father and husband
Season two, *Milkshakes for Marleigh* podcast
Adam Cheyne is incredibly grateful to Australian blood donors who saved his life after his 'life-threatening nose job'. At the age of nineteen, Adam underwent a medically necessary rhinoplasty procedure. The complications that followed were life-threating but resolved by blood transfusion.

Today, Adam is a well-respected member of his local community where he volunteers his time to ensure that there are public spaces that can be enjoyed by all. He takes greatest pride in his role as a husband and father. He thanks the blood donors who gave him the gift of life.

Rylah Joy – Model and dancer, rocking life with T21/Down syndrome
Season two, *Milkshakes for Marleigh* podcast
Rylah Joy was born prematurely and 'rode on the wings of angels and prayers' and the generosity of Australian blood donors when she overcame complications associated with her premature birth and duodenal atresia.

Rylah is now shaking up the cultural stereotypes about trisomy 21. She can typically be found on a stage or catwalk or signing deals to be a brand representative.

Baxter and Jeff – A blood donor and his possible recipient
Season two, *Milkshakes for Marleigh* podcast
Baxter was eleven months old when he was diagnosed with acute myeloid leukaemia. He is now completing his final year of schooling, is a leader in his school and local community, travelling the

world and has just accepted an offer to study at Sunshine Coast University. He knows that he owes his survival to the Australian blood donors who saved his life before he'd even celebrated his first birthday.

As Baxter was receiving his treatment in Brisbane, Jeff Steele was regularly donating platelets on the Sunshine Coast and there is a good chance that they made their way to the oncology ward of the Queensland Children's Hospital. Jeff has now made over five hundred donations, saving over 1,500 lives and keeping the same number of families together.

David Mead – Former Brisbane Bronco and former captain, Papua New Guinea, Kamuls
Season two, *Milkshakes for Marleigh* podcast

David has seen friends' babies need blood products to survive and his son spent time in a neonatal intensive care unit following his premature birth. In his retirement from being a professional athlete he is championing the need for blood donation and he is a proud member of the Milkshakes for Marleigh community.

Kylie Miller – Author and blood product recipient
Season two, *Milkshakes for Marleigh* podcast

Kylie Miller will be dependent on IVIG for life to treat multifocal motor neuropathy. She has experienced the reality of not being able access her treatment due to critical blood shortages.

Kylie is an award-winning author who has written books that have supported children through challenges such as the aftermath of the Australian bushfires of the 2019-20 summer.

Rebecca Ind – Blood donor and blood product recipient
Season two, *Milkshakes for Marleigh* **podcast**
Australian blood donors helped Rebecca Ind become a mother. After suffering recurrent pregnancy loss, she received anti-D immunoglobulin to assist her in sustaining a pregnancy and create her family.

Long before becoming a recipient, Beck was a committed long-term blood donor. She has made over two hundred donations and has no intentions of slowing down anytime soon.

Beck is the greatest cheerleader for the Milkshakes for Marleigh blood donation advocacy movement and is one of Marleigh's favourite people.

Dean Hewitt – Curler, Australian Winter Olympian
Season two, *Milkshakes for Marleigh* **podcast**
Dean thanks Australian blood donors for donating the blood that his beloved teammate and coach Ian 'Icenut' Pellagio needed while fighting blood cancer. Dean knows that the blood products Ian received gifted him more time with his loved ones and the Australian and international curling communities.

Cody and Lulu – Aussie teen achieving great things with his service dog, Lulu, by his side
Season two, *Milkshakes for Marleigh* **podcast**
Australian blood donors saved Cody's life when he was two years old and required eleven surgeries to remove a tumour in his brain. He has also trialled IVIG in an attempt treat his uncontrollable seizures.

Cody is now seventeen and working in hospitality. He has

found a great skill in creating new and innovative dishes. In 2023, he was thrilled to see his beloved team, the Collingwood Magpies, win the AFL Grand Final, with service dog, Lulu, by his side.

Cherie Canning – Founder of Luminate Leadership and host of the *Courage to Lead* podcast
Season two, *Milkshakes for Marleigh* podcast
Cherie and Andy Canning's daughter, Chloe, turns seven in 2023 thanks to Australian blood donors. Chloe was born 101 days before her due date at just twenty-five weeks gestation. She weighed just 0.73kg. Tiny Chloe was prescribed a platelet transfusion at birth to support her survival.

Today, you can find Chloe jet-setting around the world with her parents, singing and dancing her way through life while dreaming of becoming an astronaut when she grows up.

Rachael Casella – Police officer (AFP), founder of Mackenzie's Mission, author and genetic carrier screening advocate
Season two, *Milkshakes for Marleigh* podcast
Rachael and her husband Johnny are blood donors. They donate in memory of their baby girl Mackenzie, who was just ten weeks old when she received the fatal diagnosis of the rare genetic neuromuscular disorder, spinal muscular atrophy (SMA). Mackenzie passed away when she was just seven months old. In her final days, she received blood products.

Through Mackenzie's Mission, Rachael is a fierce advocate for genetic carrier screening and for ensuring that prospective parents are provided with information and choices in their family planning. She is a proud Milkshakes for Marleigh community member.

Siohhan Wilson – Fourteen-year-old business owner and blood recipient
Season three, *Milkshakes for Marleigh* podcast
Siobhan was born more than three months early and her life was saved by Australian blood donors on many occasions throughout her complex medical journey. Her mother Fiona received lifesaving blood products after the birth of Siobhan's older sister, making it possible for Siobhan to even exist!

At the age of fourteen, Siobhan is the founder of Our Pixie Friends and is on a mission to help sick kids feel less alone. She uses her lived experiences to create support packs, sensory toys and picture books to support young people all over Australia who are facing challenges or trauma.

Siobhan and Fiona thank those who donated the blood that saved their lives and encourage all eligible Aussies to consider making a donation in the future.

Molly Dawson – Blood recipient and cancer survivor
Milkshakes for Marleigh community member
Molly Dawson was seventeen and just about to commence a gap year after finishing school when she was diagnosed with Hodgkin's lymphoma. This meant relocating to Brisbane as her hometown of Bundaberg didn't have the facilities she required for treatment. While her peers were travelling the world, starting university or their careers and falling in love, Molly was undergoing gruelling chemotherapy, losing her hair and wondering if

she was going to survive.

Molly thanks Australian blood donors for making her treatment possible and giving her a future beyond cancer. She is now studying criminology at Sunshine Coast University, works at Australia Zoo and has devoted herself to volunteering and telling her story to help others. Some of her proudest moments have been working with the Sony Foundation to help young people in need, raising awareness and funds for cancer research as an ambassador for Relay for Life, offering peer support to other young people with cancer as an ambassador for Canteen's Bandana Day and being a proud blood donation advocate volunteering to tell her story to support Lifeblood in recruiting new blood donors. She is also a proud member of the Milkshakes for Marleigh community and encourages all eligible Australians to make a blood donation.

Sam Ryan – Motor vehicle accident survivor and blood donor
Milkshakes for Marleigh community member

Sam was driving from Canberra to Forbes, NSW, to work at a music festival when a microsleep resulted in his car leaving the road and hitting a tree at 100km/hour. Sam was only seventeen when he survived this near-death experience. He received large volumes of plasma and blood, which in addition to saving his life, resulted in him developing an extremely rare antibody called anti-D.

Sam is now one of the one hundred anti-D plasma donors in Australia; these antibodies save thousands of Australian babies per year. Sam knows that Australian blood donors saved his life, and he has made a lifelong commitment to blood donation in his second chance at life.

Brooke Hanson, OAM – Olympic gold medalist swimmer, former world record holder and world champion
Milkshakes for Marleigh community member
Brooke Hanson will always be known as an outstanding Australian swimmer. She is now one of Australia's most sought-after keynote speakers. Her life experience informs her work not from just her time in the pool, but in the neonatal intensive care unit (NICU), after giving birth to her son, Jack Hanson Clarke, at just twenty-eight weeks and five days, twelve weeks prematurely.

During his time in the NICU, Jack received countless blood products to sustain his life. Brooke describes that in the time she and husband Jared spent with him, Jack showed so much personality and determination. In the end, no amount of blood products could overcome Jack's chronic lung disease and pulmonary hypertension, and he lost his battle after suffering a cardiac arrest at just nine months old.

Over a decade since Jack's passing, Brooke and Jared remain dedicated to increasing awareness about premature birth, blood donation and 'the importance of family'.

Hedley Thomas – Creator of *The Teacher's Pet* podcast and journalist
Milkshakes for Marleigh community member
Hedley Thomas is one of Australia's most respected print journalists and is also responsible for the creation of Australia's most successful podcast series, *The Teacher's Pet*, which launched the medium of podcasting into the consciousness of millions of Australian listeners. It led to the reopening of the case

investigating the disappearance of Lynette Dawson and the conviction of Christopher Dawson for her murder. Hedley followed the prosecution of this case through *The Teacher's Trial* podcast, teamed with his colleagues from *The Australian*, Claire Harvey and Matthew Condon. Their assistance was required as Hedley was not able to attend the first parts of the Dawson trial due to being called as a witness.

Hedley is also responsible for the remarkable *Shandee's Story* and *Shandee's Legacy* podcasts which first aimed to investigate the murder of young Queensland woman Shandee Blackburn, but in addition resulted in the uncovering of the catastrophic failure of forensic laboratories in Queensland, resulting in The Commission of Inquiry into Forensic DNA Testing in Queensland.

When Hedley was my guest on the *Milkshakes for Marleigh* podcast, I thanked him for inspiring me to tell the stories of blood donors and their recipients in podcast format, as through listening to his work, I had seen the incredible power in the connection that could be created between a host, their guests and the audience.

Hedley: 'Podcasts create such intimacy because of the very personal connections you form with the people being interviewed. It's the honesty that you get from listening to voices without distraction. It's like a theatre of the mind.'

When I interviewed Hedley, he popped up onto the Zoom screen, hair a bit scruffy and against the backdrop of one of his children's bedrooms. He explained that he recorded most of his audio from this spare room in his house and his generosity in sharing that fact was so empowering for me going forward. My husband Geoff and I make the whole podcast; he is responsible for audio production, but I do everything else. There is no studio, no producers, nobody sources my guests or books my interviews or uploads the episodes to the host sites. Just me, my laptop and a microphone. Desperate to never again be told that Marleigh was not able to access the treatment that was preserving her life, due to blood shortages. And never wanting another Australian family to feel that fear. But watching Hedley on the screen that day, I knew that if he could make the world's biggest podcast from his daughter's bedroom, then I could make a difference from our family loungeroom.

We chatted about the unique ability of podcasts to create community and connection, engaging and mobilising listeners towards a common identity or goal. As well as the versatility of the way it way it can be consumed. Unlike the written medium, you can multitask while taking in a podcast. You can listen while driving your car, mowing the lawn or my favourite time is when I'm putting washing on the line.

Podcasts are easy to download and listen to anywhere in the world, and my message of the importance of blood donation is universal. This became apparent to me when I was advised that I was a finalist in the Women Changing the World Awards, London, 2023. I was the only Australian finalist in my category and took out the bronze award, Emerging Woman of the Year. In August 2023, I took out two silver awards in the People's Choice, Making a Difference categories of the AusMumreneur Awards, for Social Enterprise and Global Brand, recognising the international reach of the *Milkshakes for Marleigh* podcast and the impact that it's having all over the world.

Hedley and I have chatted about the great privilege of being trusted with the stories that people share with us, especially given the fear, trauma and sense of hopelessness that many of our podcast guests have endured.

Hedley: 'You need to have a connection to the people who you are narrating about or the people that you are talking to in order to appreciate it. You wouldn't want someone making a story about your life, your pain or suffering, without them being appropriately respectful or compassionate. You need to be able to put yourself in the shoes of the people that you are writing or talking about.'

In his masterful way, Hedley so beautifully describes in the quote above why Milkshakes for Marleigh is more than an Instagram page, a website, a podcast or this book: it's a community of people connected by the common goal of thanking or encouraging blood donors. He is a great supporter of my blood donation advocacy work and a proud member of the Milkshakes for Marleigh community.

Callan Ward – GWS Giants, 'best mate to Marleigh'
Proud Milkshakes for Marleigh community member
Callan has provided unwavering support, kindness and friendship to the whole Fisher family. He has been a proud supporter of the Milkshakes for Marleigh community and applauds the impact it's having on blood donation rates in Australia and around the world. Every time he kicks a goal for the GWS Giants, Marleigh cheers and tells everyone in the room, 'I bet Callan kicked that one for me!'

Libby Trickett – Olympic champion swimmer, author, podcast host, founder of Play On Media and Unlocking Her Potential, Season Two, M4M Podcast
Milkshakes for Marleigh community member
Libby has been instrumental in helping further my messages of blood donation advocacy through the *Milkshakes for Marleigh* podcast. Whether it's been through words of advice and encouragement, pointing me in the direction of Strozkiy Media, sharing a post on social media or making me laugh, a lot and often, with her Unlocking Her Potential business partner, Paula Hindle, by her side.

Lib has inspired me so much and is a strong ally in my blood donation advocacy. She is a proud Milkshakes for Marleigh community member.

Holly Wainwright – Author and podcast host, Mamamia Out Loud
Milkshakes for Marleigh community member
Holly showed extraordinary kindness to Marleigh and our family by travelling to Canberra to be the master of ceremonies for Marleigh's charity ball in November 2019. She's been generous in her encouragement of me 'finding my voice' and some of the earlier pitches of what this book may have been. I adore her pragmatism, thank her for introducing me to the musical *Hamilton*, enjoy her niche country gardening content and live in eternal envy of her podcasting and writing she-shed!

ACKNOWLEDGEMENTS

Thank you to every person featured in this book who has trusted me with telling your story. This is a privilege that I will never take for granted. Everyone featured in this book and on the *Milkshakes for Marleigh* podcast has made an incredible impact on blood donation advocacy.

If you donate blood in Australia, please ask for your donation to be added to the Milkshakes for Marleigh Lifeblood team! It's such a joy to track the number of lives saved by donors who have been inspired by the work of Milkshakes for Marleigh. Special mention to Michael Weaver for being our original and top donor! How special that first strawberry milkshake you had with Marleigh was!

To Geoff, Thomas, Campbell, Benjamin, Marleigh and Paddy – I love you all the most!

To Mum, Jake, Suz, Evie, Abbie, Jess, Matt, Molly, Billy – you are my favourite people to be with. Thanks for riding the roller-coaster with us x

To Nic, Emma, Ness, Andre, Ella, Katie, Bec, Jeff, Fran, Lisa, Sue and Vic – in no particular order. You know why x x

To Tara, Kylie, Candy – thanks for being my people.

And to Peace, Katy and the whole AusMum crew (with special mentions to Sarah and Stacey) and my amazing publisher Karen, thanks for helping me to make this big dream of mine a reality!

And as always, I will leave the final words to Marleigh: 'Thank you for my plasma!'